More *than* Enough

My Breast Cancer Story

Sherri Hildebrandt

MORE THAN ENOUGH

Front cover and headshot photography by Jessica Penner of Blackout Photography. Front cover editing by Aaron Hildebrandt and Tim Kroeker. Editing by Laurie Schellenberg and Lindsay Wright.

ISBN: 978-1-77069-220-6

Printed in Canada.

Word Alive Press
131 Cordite Road, Winnipeg, MB R3W 1S1
www.wordalivepress.ca

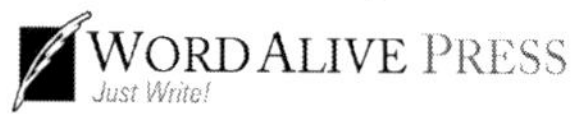

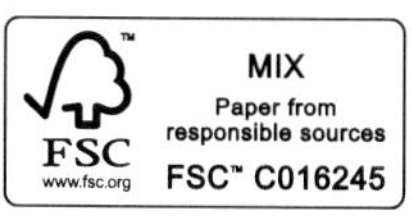

Library and Archives Canada Cataloguing in Publication

Hildebrandt, Sherri, 1959-
More than enough / Sherri Hildebrandt.

ISBN 978-1-77069-220-6

1. Hildebrandt, Sherri, 1959-. 2. Breast--Cancer--Patients--Canada--Biography. 3. Breast--Cancer--Patients--Religious life. I. Title.

RC280.B8H56 2010 362.196'994490092 C2010-907891-8

More than Enough *is dedicated first to my husband Ron. Thank you for being there through it all.*

And secondly, to my family—Lindsay, Geoff and Briony, Aaron and Caitlin, Jessica, Kevin and Chloe.

You were my motivation and inspiration to keep going forward during those times when all I wanted to do was sit down and give up.

More than enough cancer, cuts, chemo and complications;
more than enough sorrow, sickness and sadness;
and more than enough strength from God, family,
friends and unsuspecting strangers to survive.

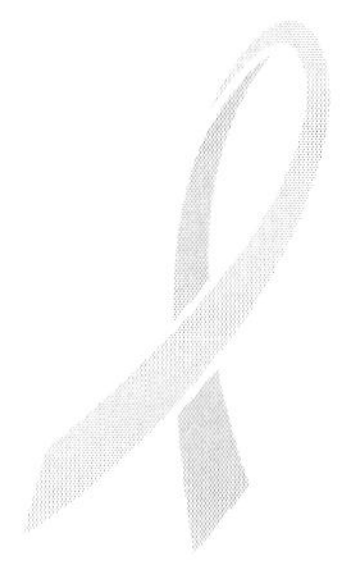

Table of Contents

Preface ix

1. In The Beginning 1

2. Surgery 15

3. Oncology 101 41

4. Chemotherapy 53

5. More Than Enough 73

6. More Chemo 81

7. Needing a Cure 99

8. Happy Thanksgiving 105

9. Same Story, Next Chapter 115

10. Radiation Therapy 119

11. Another Baby! 125

12. Ode to Joy 135

13. Decisions, Decisions 147

14. One Last Thing... 151

15. Am I a Survivor? 159

16. Say It Isn't So 163

17. On Appreciating Life 175

18. Moving Ahead 177

19. Being the Mother of a Cancer Patient 183

20. Being the Daughter of a Cancer Patient 189

21. Joy in the Journey 211

22. I'm Not Ready 217

Epilogue 221

Acknowledgements 225

Preface

I know now that everyone has their own unique story, and mine isn't special except that it's mine. And I'm convinced God told me to tell it. If you're reading it, it's either because you know me and want to relive all of the gory details, or your life has been affected by cancer in some way. Maybe you're just curious—that's okay, too. I want to be perfectly candid in saying I'm an ordinary person but I've been through an extraordinary experience. If sharing my story can help to encourage you along whatever journey you are muddling through, then it has done its job.

Chapter One
In The Beginning

I found the lump.

This answers one of the first questions people usually ask. I had been obsessively checking my breasts for any sign of a lump. A close cousin, who was only forty–seven, died in January 2008 after a courageous fight with inflammatory breast cancer. She passed away with unwavering hope and trust in God's ultimate healing. I was forty–eight years–old. This was all too close to home for me. Well, I found one at the end of that month, but concluded any lumps I had ever found in the past had resolved themselves after my menstrual cycle, so I decided to wait.

After a few weeks, I realized it was still there and it was time to check it out. I saw my family doctor February 25, and he sent me for a mammogram. He told me if he had been doing a breast exam he would never have found it, because it was so small. He was so encouraging, and gave me a wonderfully false sense of triviality. He said it was so small it could just be "scooped out," and I might need a bit of chemotherapy, but some people don't even lose their hair anymore. He made it sound so simple, and told me if it turned out to be cancer, I would probably be done treatment in a few months. My reaction, looking back now, was an unreal sense of wellbeing, because the reality of my journey was much different than the scenario he painted for me.

At the mammogram on March 5, the radiologist said the same thing about how small it was and marked the lump so she would be able to find it on the x–ray. When the results came back on March 11, the receptionist called me at 9:00 in the morning and said the doctor wanted to see me that day if possible. I waited until 4:30—my own private rebellion. I immediately thought it can't be a good sign if the doctor is asking to see you instead of the other way around! This time, I took my husband with me. I didn't want to hear the results on my own. We were informed the lump appeared to be cancerous and would need further investigation. It contained calcium flecks, which apparently is evidence of cancer. The doctor then told us I would be meeting with a surgeon who specializes in breast surgery the very next day. But, he said, don't worry about it. Every woman he has sent to this surgeon with probable breast cancer has lived. I should have asked for stats!

We met with the surgeon the next afternoon. She took the time to explain what the results of the mammogram meant, and how we would be proceeding. A biopsy was scheduled for the following day at the hospital. At this point, I was still in shock and denial. I was thinking, "This can't be happening. Is this really me they are talking about? So she does a biopsy—it can still be negative, can't it? And even if it is cancer, it can be, as the family doctor stated so eloquently, 'scooped out' and this will all be over?" Oh, if only it was that easy.

How to Spread the News 101

The beginnings of my email support team

Nowhere in the mounds of cancer material had I found any information or advice on how to talk to my young adult children about what was going on. I wasn't sure when to inform them or what should be said. I didn't want them to worry needlessly, but I also didn't want them to feel like I had excluded them from pretty important family matters. So I spoke to each of them on the phone and let them know what had transpired so far, and said nothing was conclusive yet but it didn't look positive. Their reactions were interesting and predictable. I have three children and they are all different and responded accordingly. The oldest cried and wanted more information, the middle one encouraged me and tried to trivialize, and the youngest couldn't believe it and didn't want to talk about it. As their mom, I wanted so much to shield them from the stress and turmoil of the storm that seemed to be heading our way.

And what about the extended family, my parents, sisters and brothers, in–laws, close friends and the church family? When do you inform them, and what do you say? So much that isn't in the manual! Kind of like all of the things you didn't find in the books when you started having children. It was at about this time I started a small email contact list. It seemed to be the most efficient way to get news to the important people in our lives and to keep people updated. This also gave me a base of people whom I knew would care for us and would uphold us in prayer. At that time, I had simply no idea that my family and I would need them so much—how this group of people would walk with us, endure with us and support us through our journey.

My first email entry to the team

Subject: A prayer request

Hi—I am writing to ask for prayer for myself. It's so much easier to ask for prayer for someone else but this time I need it. I found a lump in my breast a few weeks ago and was hoping it would just go away but it didn't. I saw the dr. and went for a mammogram last week. The results came in yesterday morning and I was called in for an appt. to see the dr. at 9 in the morning. I was a bit stubborn and didn't want to go, so I took a 4:30 appt. so I could go to school and stay in denial a bit longer. Ron came with me. The dr. told us that the lump has cancer characteristics and I am slated for a biopsy tomorrow morning. It is a small lump but he is concerned and that is why this is moving so quickly. I am basically calm but feel terrified underneath if you know what I mean. I told my kids, sisters and parents yesterday. Please pray for peace to prevail, and especially that this won't be cancer.

Thanks,
Sherri

Background Information

I am one of you. I am a wife, mother, working woman, and girlfriend extraordinaire. I enjoy music, reading, movies, the sound of the ocean and fighting injustice. I love making meaningful, heart–to–heart contact with people and get bored with everyday chitchat. I'm a bit short and a bit pudgy. Is this starting to sound like a cheap matchmaking bio? Don't worry, I don't want you to date me—I just want you to know I am one of you.

My husband, Ron, is pretty normal, too. Except his heart of gold shines in his eyes. He has the most annoying habit of wanting to help anyone who needs it—anytime, anywhere. He can fix anything and solve everyone's problems. I've come to realize it was really hard on him when he couldn't fix me.

We were married young and our first child was born when I was twenty–one. I say we grew up with her, and had so much fun in the process. Lindsay was a gorgeous, blonde, blue–eyed doll who talked way too soon and has honed her skills to become a communication specialist. When Lindsay was ten, she became very sick and was diagnosed with Juvenile Rheumatoid Arthritis, which has played a role in shaping her compassionate personality. She is the academic in our family, with an insatiable need to keep learning.

Lindsay was two–and–a–half when her brother Aaron came along. Being three weeks early brought challenges, and my mother came to take night shifts when he was a newborn. By the age of three, he was building robber traps in the trees to catch neighbours walking down the sidewalk. By five, he was figuring out how to program bubbles on the Commodore 64, and writing stories. He has evolved into a 3D computer animation designer and is thriving in this digital multimedia industry.

We knew from the time she was a toddler our baby Jessica was inclined to do her own thing. She was our happy–go–lucky child, who could amuse herself with an empty pizza box for hours. As a teenager, she and a friend declared a random day in spring should be "Un–Halloween Day," and dressed in costumes to go to school. Jess' creativeness and self–expression touches every aspect of her life. Her home is decorated with her photography and paintings.

Most of the children's growing–up years took place on a three–acre lot just outside of the big city. Ron commuted to work every day, and the bus came to pick up the kids for school. By the time Jessica went off to kindergarten, I had managed to graduate from university with my Educational Assistant Diploma and landed a job in the school system.

Working in Junior High Resource was a dream job. I loved building relationships with the teenagers I worked with and the ensuing joy when that friendship results in a safe, happy environment where learning is fostered. My wacky sense of humour seemed to fit the culture of the middle years, and cracked the facade of some pretty tough kids.

At the time I found the lump in my breast, I was a full–time student working on my Human Resource Management certificate at a local community college. I had made a dramatic shift in the career path I had been on for thirteen years, and wanted to explore a different direction in my working world. Now I was worrying and wondering how I would fit cancer into my busy school schedule. With all of the doctor's appointments and possible surgery, how would I be able to finish school—or would I? This tormented me, because I couldn't understand why God would lead me into quitting my stable, secure job with excellent health benefits, guide me headlong into full–time studies and then sideline me just before I would graduate and land that dream job as an HR professional. Why? He had been guiding and directing the entire past year, with losing my position at one school and transferring to another. That was when I realized I was finished with being an educational assistant and wanted something different.

The college was absolutely terrific about accommodating my cancer diagnosis and all it would involve. The instructors and friends I made during my time there were so supportive. I was able to do my presentations early, hand in assignments early and even write my exams early so I was ready to close that chapter and focus on battling cancer. On my last day at the school, my classmates and an instructor had a party for me and presented me with thoughtful gifts, including a cuddly teddy bear with "Faith" embroidered on its paw.

Email to a friend

Subject: What does this mean for school?

I talked to one of my instructors today just to let him know that I wouldn't be in tomorrow because of having a biopsy done, and I didn't know what the next little while would mean for me. He told me to not worry about school and to concentrate on myself. He said that he wasn't a religious man but he would pray for me! And he gave me a big hug with tears in his eyes. I wasn't expecting that.

I'm more scared today than I was yesterday. I don't want this. I don't like not being in control of my life.

Love,
Sherri

The Initial Biopsy

The biopsy was not what I thought it would be. It took place in the Operating Room of the Day Surgery unit of the hospital. I had no idea then that I would be back there often enough that the nurses would start to recognize me. I was very calm and even joked with the OR people. It was the middle of the annual Manitoba curling bonspiel, and I remember discussing some of the leading rinks with the nurses in the room—including opinions about one of the skips having a shiny plastic top of his head after brain surgery. A local freezing agent was administered and the fun began. The surgeon told me she would make an incision and then use a rather big needle to take out a small section of the tumour—three times. The incision was made and I didn't feel a thing. So far so good, but then one of the nurses grabbed my other arm and held it down. I wondered why. I heard a sound like two curling rocks smashing together and felt intense pressure and burning pain in my breast. My first instinct was to flail my other arm and bat away whatever was causing the pain, which was, of course, why my arm was being held down. The surgeon said, "Oh, the freezing only affects the top skin layer, not what is underneath." This happened another two times and then I was given a tissue to wipe my tears. I didn't really cry—just leaky eyes. I was proud of myself for being so brave.

I got myself dressed, walked out of there, met Ron in the waiting room and said, "Let's get out of here." I was fine until we got into the vehicle, and then I cried a bit and said, "Wow, that hurt a lot more than I had expected it to." My chest was burning and every bump in the road reminded me of what had happened in the OR.

When we got home, I grabbed that infamous bag of frozen peas and took some pain medication and the pain soon subsided. I thought I felt well enough to attend my evening class that night, and I was stubborn enough to think I could be in control and not let this take over my life. I'm not sure why I thought it was so important. I think I was craving normalcy. Cancer has a way of stealing your control, because everything is centred around the treatment and the rest of your life can seem inconsequential. By attending my evening class that night, I was trying to tell myself this won't be happening and I would continue my life as usual. Some would call it perseverance. Others stubbornness. Halfway through the evening, I called it stupid. I couldn't concentrate and my breast and arm were throbbing. But I still felt like I had accomplished something by attending and not losing my five marks for not showing up! Crazy woman!

Email to a friend

Subject: Thanks for asking...

Hey Bro...

I had my boob cut open yesterday and 3 samples taken. Other than that and feeling terrified because the doctors haven't given me much hope at all that this isn't cancer. I would like to say everything's good and it's all okay and all that, but this morning I'm not feeling that way at all and it's going to be a very long weekend waiting for the results. And trying to figure out what my life will look like once those results come back. How do you go back to school and concentrate on studying when you don't even know if you'll get to finish or even practice your new career? I know that sounds like a drama queen, but I think it might be reality according to the surgeon.

This is a new day and God will give me the strength to face it and live it to the fullest. So here I go...

I'm aiming to go for my 10:45 class this morning.

Thanks for asking,

Keep praying, please.

Sherri

Email to a friend

Subject: Hi from Sherri

The biopsy yesterday was quite painful but nothing compared to the agony of not knowing what I'm dealing with. Thank you for the words of scripture. I'm hanging on to Psalm 23 and my life verse that I've given to others many times: "May the God of hope fill you with all joy and peace, as you trust in Him, so that you may overflow with hope by the power of the Holy Spirit." (Romans 15:13, NIV)

My sister–in–law brought two vases full of daffodils on Wed. and they opened up during the night so this morning they were smiling at me when I walked into the dining room.

The Results

a.k.a The Bad News…

Email to my team

Subject: The latest news…

Hey everybody—I was informed this morning that I have an appt. for 2:30 tomorrow afternoon to see the surgeon and go over my test results.

Thank you so much for all of your prayers. I feel pretty strong considering, and I know it's the prayers. I have my moments, of course, but God shows me in many ways that He is with me so I'm trying to trust Him and lean on Him.

I've decided to go to school for the day because it doesn't do me any good to sit here by myself. That's when I lose it.

Thanks again.

We'll let you know how it turns out.

Sherri

The surgeon's office called March 20 for us to come in to speak to the surgeon. She had warned us she would not be giving results over the phone if they weren't favourable, so just having the office call us was already confirmation we were dealing with cancer. When we walked into her waiting room, we realized there were no other patients around and it was quiet. She sat on the examining table as she told us it was definitely cancer and explained the results to us. It was in an early stage and was very treatable. This was all good news to cushion the harsh reality of the "C" word. We walked out of there actually relieved to finally have confirmation and a date for surgery to remove the lump that was causing all of this fear and disruption in our lives. It felt surreal. I don't think I had ever really understood that word until then.

We walked over to the Tim Hortons beside the clinic and ordered some coffee. Ron got out his cell phone, because we knew the kids would be waiting to hear the results. I didn't feel stable enough emotionally to make the calls. His first call was to our son. Our oldest daughter Lindsay's line was busy, and we knew she was probably watching her clock at work and worrying more with every passing minute. We found out later she was texting back and forth to Aaron, who was at work himself wondering if she had heard anything yet. After those two calls, it was quite obvious we were making a scene in the coffee shop, so we decided to continue outside where we could lose our dignity in private. Tears flowed freely as we talked to our youngest, Jessica, while walking back to our vehicle at the clinic.

The strangest thing is I remember the sun was shining brightly and it felt warm, like an embrace. There wasn't panic—just a profound disappointment that what we had feared was really true. Life would be very different and difficult for the next while. We didn't even entertain thoughts of death. We just couldn't go there. The doctor told us it was a good prognosis, which meant to us that I would need surgery and then possibly chemo and radiation. That's what we told our children. And that's what we were clinging to.

Unexpected

a.k.a The Good News…

By the weekend, we knew it was important to rally our family. In the past year, our tightly knit group of five had miraculously and quickly grown to eight. We were all learning how to relate as a bigger group, and our new expanded family was really becoming a lot of fun. The oldest and youngest, both girls, were both newly married, and our middle son had a rock–solid, steady relationship with a girl we loved and accepted as one of our own. So we invited everyone home for a family dinner on Sunday to regroup, process and commiserate together. Little did we know what that evening had in store. Remember, this is good news, so you can keep reading.

At the dinner table that Sunday evening, my oldest daughter handed me a card. On the front it said, "I guess what you need right about now is a great big…" and inside, in her writing, "How about a grandchild?" When things settled down a bit, Lindsay told us that on the very same day we saw the doctor for the results of my mammogram, she had been at the same doctor an hour later getting the results from her pregnancy test. She was on birth control and had no idea she was pregnant, so this was a huge and unexpected event in their lives. They had only been married for five months and weren't planning to have children for quite a while yet.

That's about when our youngest daughter, Jessica, presented us with another gift bag. This one held some baby bibs that said, "If Mommy says no…ask Grandma." Lindsay looked puzzled and Geoff, her husband, asked Jessie, "How did you know?" He was thinking someone had guessed about their pregnancy or spilled the news about them.

All of a sudden, Lindsay caught on and explained to

Geoff. "She's pregnant too!"

I ran to the kitchen window, trying to get my emotions under control. I remember loud, gasping, ugly sobs coming out of me and tears springing up from deep down inside and overflowing. My grown–up children sat at the table watching helplessly. Ron came from behind and wrapped his arms around me. I finally got my emotions under control and tried to explain these were happy tears. It was just such an intense roller coaster of emotions.

I need to confess that Ron and I already knew about the news our youngest daughter and her husband had shared. She lives close by and came over one evening a few weeks earlier with a small gift bag and presented it to me. In it was a thermometer—at least that's what I thought it was at first. Then, silly me—it dawned on me that it was a pregnancy tester and it read positive! I think I yelled out loud. She was so young and they had been married just over a year. Her doctor had advised her that if they were planning to have children, she would need to go off her method of injections for birth control because it could take two years for it to get out of her system. They decided to discontinue the injections, and 'voila!'—a baby was conceived in the first month. So we knew about this and we were thrilled and excited at the prospect of becoming grandparents. I knew they would be very good parents, and the unexpected news didn't seem to faze them.

I'm so glad I knew about Jessica and Kevin's announcement, because by this time I couldn't take much more excitement. I enjoyed the two girls realizing their due dates were just a bit more than a week apart. What a God moment. I can imagine His delight as His orchestrated plan came together. This was a very unexpected but most awesome, thrilling and exciting turn of events at a time in my life when God knew what I needed to give me the motivation to beat the disease that had just begun to invade my life and threaten to take away my joy of living.

Grandma. I have loved the notion of being a grandma ever since I had my own babies—thinking that someday I would love to be a grandma and how much I would enjoy and treasure grandbabies in my arms. Lindsay informed her father that she didn't think she would let her child near him until the child was old enough to say, "Grandpa is crazy." I *think* she was joking!

Email to my children

Subject: So…now what?

I just want to tell all of you that I was dreading tonight. I didn't want it to be a cry fest but my heart was breaking trying to figure out how to handle my feelings. I needed to be with my kids and hug them. There is no manual that I'm aware of that tells you how to deal with this. I want to be strong for you and yet my own emotions are running rampant. But WOW—I can't believe that God is turning this into such a wild ride. I am so incredibly overwhelmed with joy and disbelief—you probably figured that out. 2 little grandbabies. Who would have believed it?

Thanks for making my day. I can't stop smiling.

Love,

Mom

Chapter Two
Surgery

First Surgery

Email to my friends at the college

Subject: My non–school test results

Well, I got my test results, and I have cancer. I feel kind of like an alcoholic having to name it at an AA meeting. I wanted to let you know, but I also want to tell you that the prognosis is good. The other testing that has been done has all come back clear which is very good. So my surgery date is set for April 8th and then treatment plans will be made according to the results of what they find. I don't know what that means for finishing school. I think if I feel I'm emotionally strong enough, I'm going to try to keep coming to school and finishing what I can before surgery. I have so many encouraging people in my life, including you—my school family—who are helping me with your encouragement and support. I'll probably see you next week. Have a good Easter.

Thanks,

Sherri H.

I thought going through one surgery would be it, and I would do the treatments needed and then I would be cancer–free. I refused to even think about the idea that there might be another plan. Sure there was that nagging fear way deep down, but I refused to give in to feeling it unless it became a reality. I was very intent on staying strong.

The Sentinel Node Injection

My surgery day started with what is called a sentinel node injection. It was to be done at St. Boniface Hospital. As we were walking from our vehicle in the hospital parking lot, we heard a shout, "Hi, Ron and Sherri!" It was a couple from our church who had just finished an appointment with a doctor there at the Cancer centre. He had been successful in fighting a cancer tumour in one of his fingers. They are on our email prayer support team, and it was very reassuring to me that God had orchestrated this "chance" meeting. This couple let us know we were being prayed for and supported every step of the way—especially today. It was kind of like a hug from God letting me know He was very aware of what I was going through and He was holding me.

So this sentinel node "injection" implied that one injection would be given to the lump site and no research I read said otherwise. What in fact transpired at that appointment was not one injection, but five in total. The doctor administering these injections asked my husband to step around to the other side of the table to hold my hand so I could squeeze it if I needed to. Uh, oh. He said some women don't find these needles painful at all, but some find them quite uncomfortable. I was so determined to be stoic. I had an army of people praying for me and I was not going to let them down at the very beginning of my surgery day. I had a long way to go yet. So I was brave and the first needle wasn't too bad. I told myself, I can do this. The second was a bit worse as the doctor progressed around the circumference of my breast. Okay, the third one was absolute torture. I suddenly pulled out my old labour breathing that had been lying latent and dusty in the recesses of my mind. After a brief break, I said let's get this over with and the next injection was done. The doctor said the last one is really just like a bee sting, so it won't really hurt. Youch! What size of Amazonian bee was that? When it was over, I asked the doctor if he had ever personally had these injections, and what made him think it felt like a bee sting if he had never actually experienced it himself—all said very politely, of course.

Note: I've done some research since I wrote this and since last spring (2009), there is a new way of doing this sentinel node injection. It's so reassuring to know headway is being made in treating breast cancer. Apparently, an anaesthetic is added to the radioactive dye that is being injected and the pain of the injection is reduced from a seven out of ten to about a two out of ten.

After the injections we had an hour to kill (oh, bad choice of words? Get used to it—if you can't learn to find the humour in all of this, you've lost the battle) before we were expected to register at the next hospital where the actual lumpectomy and sentinel node removal would take place. Ron had a great idea. We stopped at a Dollar Store and specifically looked for things we might possibly need for camping the next summer—our retreat at the Falcon Lake seasonal camping site we "won" through the lucky lottery system for the third year in a row. This stop was a very good distraction, and we made some wise purchases as we sauntered through the store in a bit of a "cancer surgery day" stupor.

The Lumpectomy

Next stop was the Victoria Hospital Day Surgery unit. I had been there before when I had the biopsy done and I knew the routine. One of the concerns I had about the pre–op activity was very legitimate. I have always had trouble with IVs (Intravenous Line), and in a medical situation I had faced a few years prior, I had endured seven attempts from various medical personnel to secure a vein to support an IV. I ended up with this IV in the crook of my arm, supported by a brace, and anyone touching me had been warned that this site was precious and not to be tampered with. I had met with the Day Surgery pre–op nurse a few days before this surgery and I was assured the anaesthetist in the OR would be starting the IV, so I didn't need to worry about it. My HR course in Assertiveness Training came in handy as I had to fight off the day surgery nurse who ushered me to my bed and supervised me changing into the happy blue gown and pretty matching "slippers."

The next thing that needed to be done was to start the IV. I said, "No. I was assured that the anaesthetist would be starting it in the OR." She grabbed my arm and said she just wanted to look at my veins. Obviously she had done this before. In a split–second, she had that rubber band choking the circulation in my arm and was feeling for the lucky vein. She was no match for me, though, and I had that rubber band off in no time. I asked her to please read my chart and she would see what I was talking about. She wasn't happy with me. I didn't care at that point. She was quiet as she perused my chart, and then just walked away, and that was the last I saw of her.

The time came and went for my surgery. All this time, I was waiting for the panicky feeling to hit. The one where it's hard to breathe, your heart is racing, and you just want to throw up or go home. As we waited, Ron worked on a Sudoku puzzle and I snuggled in the bed and almost fell asleep. I knew it was God. He had heard the prayers of the people supporting us and had given us that peace that passes understanding. When the surgeon finally came to see us before the surgery, it had already been delayed by over an hour. But it was all good. After talking with her again, I was sure I could trust her and would be safe in her hands. She explained exactly what would be taking place in the operation and reminded us she would be injecting blue dye to find the sentinel nodes, so I would be looking bluish after it was over. Ron liked that part and called me his "little Smurfette." I was rolled into the OR and the anaesthetist was waiting for me. He managed to put that IV in with one try—albeit with everyone else standing around waiting for him. He looked at me and said, "I'm only going to do this once and I'm going to do it right." The doctor and nurses in the room were discussing the new nursing contract and I was talking to them about being a union steward. I was enjoying the discussion. The next thing I knew I woke up and I had another point to make about the contract discussion, but no one was around. It took me a minute to realize where I was and that the discussion had probably finished without me a few hours ago.

I was wheeled back to my day surgery unit and my husband, who was sitting there waiting for me. I don't remember much about the rest of that evening. I returned from surgery around 6:00 and at 9:00, I was strongly encouraged to sit up and eat and drink and be merry. I remember thinking I was not in any shape to go home yet. I hadn't even peed yet—don't you always need to show them you are capable of peeing before they send you on your way? But the day surgery closed at 9:30 and everybody had to go home no matter what shape they were in, even if surgery had been delayed. Somehow the gown came off, my clothes were put on and I was plopped down into a wheelchair. A nurse wheeled me out to the hospital entrance as my husband went to get the car. She stayed with me waiting for him and confessed, "I can't believe they are sending you home. They never would have done this five years ago. I can't believe it." She wiped tears from her eyes. I don't think my husband could believe it, either. I made it into the house with his help and crashed on the sofa. He took a picture of me that night so others could appreciate the blue hue of my skin. My fondest memory of that surgery day was that the new, mauve, button–up shirt I had purchased for this solemn occasion matched the walls of the day surgery unit. I didn't know then that I would be wearing it again.

Email update to my team

Subject: Update on Sherri

Thank you for your prayers. They were felt and appreciated.

Sherri's surgery was two hours long. It started a bit late so she wasn't back to day surgery till six and we were not able to get home till 10:30 last night. She was very well taken care of and experienced no nausea after. This was a real answer to prayer. Because of previous blood clots, and a family history, I had to take her back to the Vic. this morning and the next two for injections to lessen the chance of this complication. This was not a pleasant trip for her. Please continue to pray for a speedy recovery, no complications and patience as we wait for results, which will be a few weeks.

Ron (and Sherri)

Recovery From Surgery Number One

Recovery from this simple lumpectomy and sentinel node removal seemed much harder than I could recall others had experienced from the research I had done. There are so many stories of women going back to work a week after the surgery. What's the deal with that? I was just barely coping with the pain and swelling when we went to see the surgeon after a week of recovery, but my condition made sense when she informed us she had "carved out a cavern." Apparently, the lump had been larger than what the mammogram had shown, so to ensure clear margins she had taken out a bigger section than she had originally planned. We had given her that freedom when we talked to her at the hospital. We let her know we were much more concerned with removing the cancer than what my breast might look like after. I wanted any and all cancer out of my body, and my husband had assured me he just wanted me healthy again. Having the surgeon tell us what had happened was like being given permission to not be up to par yet—the pain and swelling were justified, and it was okay not to have bounced back like the other superwomen I had heard and read about.

EMAIL UPDATE TO MY TEAM

I thought I would take a minute out of my busy day—sleeping, drinking tea, sleeping again, going for a walk, sleeping again... to say a huge thanks to you for keeping me in your prayers. Surgery is behind me and I feel like every day is another step toward wellness. The pain is tolerable and I have found that I am needing drugs less today than yesterday. I had a shower today and if you've never had surgery it might seem silly but it is incredible to feel clean again! I don't think I'll go into details about surgery but I think it went well, and my blood–thinner shots are done as of yesterday so that means no complications! Yay! I am overwhelmed and humbled by the love and support you have shown me and Ron and my family. Words can't express how grateful I am that I'm not doing this by myself. You've asked what the next step is and that would be waiting...again... We are waiting for the results of all of the testing of the tumour and lymph nodes. The results will determine my treatment plan. My next appt. is with the surgeon on the 21st.

So thanks again for your friendship and support. Your prayers sustained us. God is good.

Love,

Sherri

EMAIL UPDATE TO MY TEAM

I had an appt. today with my surgeon for my follow–up. We were expecting results of the testing today, too. I heard the details of the surgery—and was informed that I was doing very well considering what she had done to me! But there were no results in yet. She said that wasn't necessarily a bad thing because if there was concern the testing would have been done faster. So she says the results should be in this week yet, and she'll give me a call. It was quite disappointing, because we want to know what exactly we are dealing with and get the treatment started. The sooner it starts, the sooner it's done, right? And my aim is to be healthy and ready to be a grandma in fall. So that's where it's at. Thanks again for all of your prayer support and encouragement. I've been feeling quite anxious since yesterday because I thought we would get the results today but now that didn't happen and the waiting game is rough—for everybody. Please pray for renewed peace and calm in the storm.

Love,

Sherri (and Ron)

I was still in recovery mode, and not even worrying so much about the results, so when the phone rang, I wasn't prepared for what I heard. I had been so thoroughly convinced I was finished with my cancer treatment. The doctor had told me the lump had probably taken between five to seven years to develop, so in my mind there would be no way it could have spread anywhere yet. The call came at seven in the evening from the surgeon. She thought we would want to know as soon as possible...one of the sentinel nodes showed traces of cancer. She was very hopeful because it was only microscopic, minute traces, and that was one of the reasons it had taken a while to get the results. It had taken a second screening of the nodes to find it. But the news was in. She had already booked the date of the next surgery to remove the rest of the lymph nodes under my affected arm—a complete axilliary dissection. She had explained the possibility of this surgery to us beforehand, but I had hardly heard her because I was so convinced I wouldn't need it. The second surgery would be even more invasive, and would require a longer recovery time. I hung up the phone, and sat there. Ron stood beside me while I tried to process. It was such a deep and profound disappointment. I honestly thought God would spare me from this.

When the realization flooded in, it hit hard. I finally collapsed in Ron's arms and shook with sobs. Scores of questions washed over me—"How could I survive another surgery so soon after the one I had just endured and was not fully recovered from? How could I tell my children, my mom, my sisters, this awful news?" Fear was rampant—"Where else has the cancer spread to? Am I dying? How long do I have? How much longer will this whole nightmare take to be over—one way or another?" And on and on.

I realized this second surgery would change the entire timeline of the next year. Treatment would be postponed until I had recovered from it. That meant I might not be finished with treatments and healthy by the time my little grandbabies would be born. I *really, really* wanted to be healthy and there for my daughters as they would be having their first babies. Doesn't every mother want to do that? Oh, it hurt. We did the only thing we knew to do in a situation so out of our control—we gave it to Jesus. It sounds so simple, but it is so profound. There are things too heavy and painful and scary for us to carry ourselves. We gave it to Jesus in prayer and, again, we experienced calmness in the storm.

I had no idea why He chose to keep me in this nightmare. I knew that at any time He could heal me completely and totally. For some higher and lofty reason, He was choosing to have me walk this path, through this particular valley. The only control I had then, and have now, is in how I choose to handle every day, every hour, every minute—in my attitude, and in my choices. Do I choose to trust Him and live every day with purpose? I'm not there yet, and I'm certainly not a saint. But I'm trying, and that's all He's asking of me.

Email update to my team

Well, we need to ask you to keep praying. The surgeon phoned tonight with the results of the surgery testing. When a dr. calls at 7:30 at night, you have a feeling this isn't going to be good. There were traces of cancer found in one of the lymph nodes. This means more surgery. I'm slated for May 6th for a complete axilliary lymph node dissection. This is not the news we wanted and were hoping and praying for. Recovery is longer and more difficult with this additional surgery, but it is necessary to determine how many lymph nodes are involved so the stage of cancer and treatment can be figured out.

We thank you for continuing to pray for us.

Sherri and Ron (and family)

By this time, I realized my little email prayer team had grown to a number I had no control over. This is the risk you encounter when you use the Internet as a medium of communication. It's efficient, but you can't realistically manage who is reading your intimate thoughts. It was time to rein in the troops and regain some measure of control, so I added this disclaimer to my latest email. I recommend doing this if you are using email to keep connected during a difficult time.

**We'd also like to request that you ask us before you forward these updates to anyone else. This is our own private group of support people and even though the extra prayer is appreciated, it's kind of creepy knowing that our personal lives are being exposed to anyone—anywhere. Also, please let us know if you don't want to be on our list of support people. We can handle that because we realize that this isn't a pleasant journey and some of you might be in a place in your lives where you don't wish to be leaned on. We made this list without asking some of you, but assuming you would want to be. Again, please let us know if you want out of this.*

The Get–Away

One of the things we have always talked about doing sometime in the future, once we retire, is to be coordinators for a mission project somewhere in a disaster area. We had decided to look for a new camper and had been dealing on one in the midst of this cancer experience. This was to be the camper we would tow with us to a work site and live in for extended periods, but for now it was going to be our retreat at the lake. The complication of this deal was that the camper was situated in Michigan, and we had been planning to go pick it up once I had recovered from my first surgery. With the second surgery looming, we had a dilemma—how and when were we going to be able to go get it? We discussed it at length and decided now was as good a time as any. It had been two weeks since surgery, and I was starting to feel much better. We borrowed our son–in–law's truck and started out.

On the first day, we made good time and by evening we were well on our way…and then we hit an April blizzard in the middle of Minnesota. This was a blizzard to write home about, and the funny thing was I don't think I thought about cancer or surgery or anything else while we were driving through the mounds of snow on the Interstate. We heard later it had been closed behind us. We finally made it through to the city we were aiming for, but only after taking two tries to locate the ramp to get into the city. It was storming so badly we couldn't make out the road signs. Thank God for GPS. It told us when a curve was coming up in the highway ahead and we were able to stay on the road by following the picture on the screen. The hotel we found for that night had mounds of snow on the parking lot and we were very glad our borrowed truck was a 4x4 and we were able to drive in and find a room.

This whole ordeal was a wonderful distraction for us and made for a great story to tell people when we got home, because there wasn't a speck of snow here. We had a good time laughing about what might have happened if we had hit the ditch. Trying to get travel insurance to leave on this trip had been a difficult experience for me because of my new diagnosis, but I had managed to secure some. But Ron bought his insurance at a different location, and he was only covered starting at midnight that night, whereas my coverage had already started. We joked about how I would need to keep the medics occupied or hide his body till after midnight, so that the insurance would have kicked in and he could get medical help.

It was a great experience meeting the couple selling the camper. God must get a kick out of connecting random people in the weirdest circumstances. Some day I'm going to ask Him about how He manages to do all of this, because I was under the misconception He was busy figuring out wars and famine and end–of–the–world stuff. I think it's crazy that He spent time on the logistics of who we would meet when we bought this camper out in Michigan. The woman who owned the camper is a nurse. Not just any nurse. She is an oncology nurse who works with the doctor who removes the port–a–cath when cancer patients are finished with their chemotherapy. She and I spent some time discussing my experiences so far, and because of her knowledge and expertise, she was able to encourage me and help to calm my fears. I felt like God knew I needed exactly this so I could face what was coming with more confidence. It was even more meaningful for us when we discovered she and her husband are passionate followers of Christ and pledged to pray for us.

I'm including the story of our trip because it had a substantial impact on my cancer journey. We picked up the camper and it was all we had hoped for. We soon realized after we started the trip homeward that towing the camper home would be a rock n' roll experience. The truck was shaking and rocking with the weight of the camper. I survived the trip by holding two pillows under and against my poor, recovering post–surgical side. By the time we finally got home, I was in so much agony!

The next morning when I woke, I felt like there was something very wrong with my affected breast. The incision site was swollen and angry, and I was very afraid it was infected. This was a complication I hadn't had yet and I wasn't very happy. As the day progressed, the children all came home for supper to say hi and, of course, to see the new camper. I tried to carry on as if everything was okay, but the pain was increasing. By the time supper was ready and we all sat down to eat, I was consumed by the pain and thought I might pass out. I lay down and Ron called the surgeon. She was on call and we left everything at home and made our way to the hospital. Lindsay sent out a quick email to my support team to ask for prayer.

EMAIL TO THE TEAM

Subject: Urgent prayer request

It's not Sherri…It's Lindsay (tricky, hey?).

Geoff and I—along with Jess and Kevin—were over at my mom and dad's place for dinner tonight, and my mom was feeling progressively worse. She developed an abscess beneath her surgical incision today, and it was growing in size. As it grew, her pain started to increase and she was fighting fainting spells from the pain.

Fortunately, her surgeon is on call tonight—so my parents left for the hospital a few minutes ago. There, they'll drain the abscess and check her out to make sure that everything is okay.

My mom asked that I email all of you, her support team, and ask you to please pray:

1. That things will go smoothly at the hospital tonight
2. That there aren't any complications (specifically, that the abscess doesn't mean there's an infection)
3. That she'll be feeling better again very soon
4. That she'll experience peace in the place of panic over this unexpected complication

I'm sure that one of my parents will be able to update everyone later tomorrow, once we know more about what's going on.

Thank you so much! I know that your love and prayers and support mean the world to her (to all of us).

Lindsay

The doctor met us at the hospital and took us straight into an examining room. She knew right away what we were dealing with and said the "cavern" was swollen with fluid and needed to be drained, but she only wanted to take a bit of fluid out so the pressure would be relieved, but the shape of the breast would not be in jeopardy. That was when she got out the biggest syringe I have ever seen in my life. I looked at Ron and he looked at me and not a word was said, but we knew what each other was thinking—Oh, my goodness!

The most amazing thing happened…the exact spot she drove the needle into was one that had no feeling in it after surgery. It honestly didn't hurt at all. And as the "little bit" of fluid filled the syringe, the pressure was relieved instantly. I had been shaking and on the verge of throwing up and passing out with the pain, and instantly it vanished and I felt so much relief. Praise the Lord. There was no sign of infection in the fluid or the incision site, and I was free to go home. I felt like hugging the doctor—I'm not sure, maybe I did. No, actually, she hugged me. She said I was doing fine, but chastised me for going on this road trip. She asked me—didn't I know I wasn't ready or recovered enough to do this? How should I have known? She assured me I had a healthy breast and that she had been as surprised about the lymph nodes being affected as I had been. But it was very reassuring to hear from her that even though I would need to endure the second surgery, she was confident the results would be good and wouldn't affect the treatment plan aside from moving it down the road. This chance meeting with the surgeon because of the fluid build–up was actually a huge blessing, because it gave us an opportunity to talk with her face–to–face and be reassured that things were going to be fine. She did make us promise to discuss any further road trips with her *before* we went. We found out later when we got back home that Lindsay had sent out the above email call for prayer and we knew without a doubt that God had heard and He had answered.

A Little Sign for Me

We attended church that next Sunday, because I was recovered enough and we felt it was time to worship with the people who were spending time on their knees on our behalf. One of the songs that had been going through my mind in the previous weeks was one we used to sing years ago in our worship services but hadn't heard for a long time. It's called "Power of Your Love." I had been wondering if I should ask for one of the bands at church to sing it as a favour for me. One of my close friends was leading worship that Sunday. Wouldn't you know it—one of the songs she had picked for that morning was exactly that song? She introduced it by saying she didn't know why, but she felt like God had impressed on her that the band needed to include this song. They had almost scrapped it during sound–check that morning because it hadn't gone well, but the Lord told her somebody needed to hear it that morning, so she obeyed and encouraged the band to do it. I told her about it after the service and she cried. I was so glad she and the band had obeyed, because it was such a blessing to me. It was like a huge banner was flying for me to see and know without a doubt that God was aware of my situation and He wanted to show me so I would know. She said she was so happy I had told her, because it gave her so much more confidence in listening to God's voice and knowing she needed to obey because of the impact it has on the people God wants to use them to minister to.

MOTHER'S DAY 2008

My Mother's Day was different. My family had become so much more affectionate and loving. I'm just sorry it takes something so drastic and scary to meld a family like this. I think the way our family had grown so quickly, with the girls becoming pregnant so unexpectedly, and now this cancer diagnosis, had enabled some fast–track bonding. My children surprised me with an extra special gift this year—an iPod. Aaron had been stealthily taking my CDs and loading them onto it. It was full of my music and some of his favourite music and books he insisted I just had to listen to!

I Don't Want to Die

A few days before my second surgery, I had a total and complete meltdown. It was scary. I had been alone all day while Ron was teaching. During the afternoon, I had a phone call from a girl from my church who had been through a lymphoma cancer experience, and we discussed everything from chemo side effects to port installation, hair loss and more. About an hour before I expected Ron home, I became anxious, distraught, full of fear, and then I felt a different level of scared—I was absolutely terrified. I started to cry and as I cried, my sobs became more pronounced and deep and scary. I was losing it and I knew it. I cried and cried and the more I tried to control it, the worse it got. I didn't want to die and I didn't want to have to go through another surgery and I didn't want to do this—any of it. I was really feeling sorry for myself. I didn't deserve this—any of it. I was scared to the core. I knew I had been trying to be strong for my husband, my children, for my own mom and dad, my sisters and everyone else, so they would think I was doing so well that they didn't need to be hurting and worrying about me. But by keeping it all in, I was actually hurting myself and my body knew it. So I cried uncontrollably, knowing Ron would be coming home to this and even though I tried to regain my composure, I just couldn't stop myself. He came in the door and all hell broke loose. He held me and I sobbed and sobbed from way down deep inside. I'm crying now as I'm writing this, because I have never experienced such deep and profound emotional agony before. It was as if I had to go down that deep to get it all out. After a while, I had no more tears and it subsided. Ron cried and prayed with me and I felt better than I had in a long time.

I think in retrospect, it was a way of relinquishing my control of my situation. I knew that whatever was still ahead on the road to recovery was necessary and unavoidable—complications included—and I needed to lean on the Lord and trust Him wholeheartedly to get through it. I also realized I needed to be more real and open and honest with others—the safe ones—if I was going to get through this, not just physically, but mentally and emotionally.

Surgery 2

Complete Axilliary Dissection

Email to my team

Subject: surgery tomorrow

To our friends and family:

Just a reminder about my upcoming surgery tomorrow morning at 7:45. Your prayers were answered for the first surgery so I won't be changing my request a lot. Thank you so much for the prayers, love and support. Here we go again…

Please pray for:

- The IV situation to go well
- No complications (blood clots)
- No infection
- Peace, strength and courage
- For the surgeon—wisdom, skill, etc.

Please also pray for Ron and for our children. The twists in the path on this journey are taking their toll on the family and they need your prayers too.

Thanks for the emails and calls we have received to let us know that you remember.

We have felt God's peace—most of the time, and know God is good, all the time.

Love,

Sherri and Ron

Email to my children

Subject: To my kids

Hey, I just want to tell you how much I love you. I don't want to go through surgery again tomorrow but I will because I want to be here for many more years to be your mom.

Dad doesn't think he needs anybody at the hospital, but if any of you want to come make sure he eats some supper—or sit with me so he feels okay about going to eat supper, that might be a good idea. I've told anybody else who asks that I don't want any company. But I've told Dad that if any of my kids shows up that would be alright with me.

So in case you don't know, I love you, I love you, I love you.

Love,

Mom

The second surgery was to remove a slab of tissue containing as many lymph nodes as possible from under my arm, using the same incision from the first surgery. The complications from this surgery could range from numbness in the back of my arm from snipping that particular nerve, to lymphedema, which is the swelling of the affected arm because the lymphatic fluid has lost its pathways and can't drain, and the arm becomes swollen and painful. I was staying overnight in the hospital after this surgery. I was glad the surgery was scheduled to be the first one in the morning so I could get it over with and not have to wait in nervous anticipation for too long, and without having to starve for too long. So I wore the same dusty mauve shirt that matched the color of the walls in the day surgery unit—hey, it seemed to work the first time—and off we went at 6:00 in the morning.

The pre–op nurse had listened this time, and no mention was made of trying to start the IV. I was informed that the master anaesthetist would be starting it in the OR and I was so relieved…until I learned he hadn't shown up for work yet. By the time I was actually in the OR and lying there, he still hadn't appeared and it seemed a slightly "less–than master" anaesthetist would attempt it. Well, I can say I was really glad he froze it before he tried, because it didn't work. I remember thinking to myself that no one outside of this room knows this isn't working. How can I let Ron know so he can pray for me? Slight panic moment. So he tried a second spot, froze it (that means another needle; ironic, eh?) and apparently it did the trick because I was out like a light. When I woke, I was in PAIN! The nurse in the recovery room informed me I was dealing with low blood pressure, so I wouldn't be given any pain killers until my blood pressure was up. I don't know how long I lay there crying quietly because it hurt too much to let myself actually wail and let 'er rip. Finally, she injected some morphine into my IV and the pain subsided. The next thing I knew I was in my hospital room and Ron was standing beside me and it wasn't even noon yet.

EMAIL UPDATE FROM RON TO THE TEAM

Thank you for your prayers and support.

From the way surgery went today, I know ***most*** of you were praying. The surgery went well, started at 7:45, done by 10:00. The surgeon said it would be a two and a half hr. "procedure".

There were a few complications:

- The IV did not cooperate, so her hand is pretty bruised up.
- Her blood pressure was very low after. It was an hour and a half before they could start her on some morphine…Sherri was ***extremely grumpy*** by then.

She was back in her room by noonish, slept, rested, ate a bit by 7ish and rejoicing and trusting there will be no more surgeries.

I hope to have Sherri home tomorrow morning.

Please pray for rest, God's peace, and good results from this last surgery.

Ron

My Hospital Story

The hospital stay itself deserves its own special section. After the first surgery, I couldn't believe they had sent me home in the state I was in and thought I would be better off in the hospital. After the second surgery, I was thinking, "Just take me home!"

I had a roommate. She was an older woman who made the most pathetic, pitiful groaning noises. She was so needy that when I used my call button, she stopped the nurses who came in and kept them occupied so they didn't remember or realize that it was ME who rang for help. Every time she moved in bed or attempted to reach something on her bedside table, she would emit these moans and groans I have yet to be able to emulate, and believe me, I've tried…thinking they might elicit more sympathy or something. It never worked for me like it did for her! I thought to myself, I have just come out of major surgery and I am very much in pain and I still can't allow myself to be so pathetic. I wanted to scream, "Just suck it up and take it like a man!" But that wouldn't have been very kind of me.

Lindsay showed up to relieve Ron so he could go find himself some supper. He came back with some French fries, and that was what sustained me because I wasn't brought any supper. We asked about it and waited some more. At about seven o'clock, I was treated to a liquid diet supper of some soup broth. I asked for some crackers to make it more of a meal. Yum.

Aaron and his girlfriend Caitlin stopped in to check on me. My roommate had a TV and just happened to be watching *American Idol*. She offered to angle the TV so we could watch it, too, but I think she was sorry she had done this because Lindsay and I had very different opinions about the contestants than she did. It was nice for her to share her TV with us, though, and it helped to distract me from my pain and made the time go faster.

At about two in the morning when I went to the bathroom, after my roommate had called for help every half–hour, and no one had slept a wink yet, I was walking back to my bed and I heard her quietly sobbing in her bed. I got to my bed and stood there for a minute. Should I talk to her? And God said, pray with her. I said no way. He said yes, she needs you. I thought, maybe it will calm her down and she will go to sleep and then maybe I can get some sleep. So even with my own selfish motives, I went over to her bed and asked, "Can I pray for you?"

She said, "What?" incredulously. I repeated it. And she said yes, I would like that. And so I did. I don't actually remember what I prayed. It was one of those prayers that you know while you're praying that the Spirit just took over and is using you as his tool to speak to the person. You have obeyed and are now ministering to this person but not in your own power. She was visibly impacted and was very appreciative, but she did not settle down at all, as I had hoped. But I felt like I done what I was supposed to do and so I was blessed and still very much awake.

About this time, I managed to scrounge around in my bag and found my iPod and put in the earbuds to drown out my roommate's groaning. I flipped to a random CD of worship songs I hadn't listened to in a while. In the darkness of that hospital room, I was ministered to by a song I had heard many times and yet had never really listened to the words. I played it once, and then again, and cried through the entire song. It was called *Stronger than the Storm* and it was just what I needed to hear. I realized again that even though I have so little actual control over what is happening to me in all of this, I know the Person who is ultimately in control, and He loves me and I can trust Him.

I also need to mention a freaky moment during the night when I opened my eyes and thought I saw an angel beside my bed. I remember thinking a really stupid thought—this would be great for the book I'll write when this is all done—and then

I realized this angel was really my IV pole, and then I remember feeling really stupid!

A nursing assistant helped me with my back brace after going to the washroom during the night. He was an older black gentleman with a Jamaican accent. He offered to bring me something to drink and came back with a glass of apple juice. I drained it quickly and he waited so he could take my glass when I was done, and then he offered to get me some more. I remembered this because he was one of the only people who wasn't preoccupied with my roommate and seemed to want to take care of me. He came back when his shift was over and told me he just wanted to wish me luck and to say I would be in his prayers. He said, "You're gonna be okay," in his Jamaican accent and it was just what I needed to hear.

When Ron came in the morning, I was more than ready to go home.

Email from Ron to our children

Subject: Da Mama

FYI: "Mama eagle has landed in her nest"

Mom had a horrible night, unable to sleep with the willy nilly commotion of hospital life, very glad to be in her own bed. We have many drugs, the world will be fine again...eventually.

Dad

Surgery 2 Recovery

Recovery was hard—made even more difficult because of the drainage tube sticking out of me. It needed to be drained often and I had trouble even looking at it, let alone trying to drain it. We were shown how to do it before we left the hospital, and Ron knew it would be his job. This was really hard for me, because it felt so humbling for me to lean on him like this. Kind of like if he would need to change my dirty diaper, except not quite that bad! He was so incredibly awesome and I remember one time he had drained the grenade–looking bulb and was stripping the tubing when an incredible pain shot into my arm—we realized later it was nerve damage from the surgery—and he actually cried because he had hurt me. Sleeping was so difficult because I could only sleep on one side and couldn't actually turn myself to find another position without help. He helped me lower myself into bed, positioned all of the pillows I needed for support, and then tucked me in so lovingly. I felt very loved and cared for. I thanked the Lord that He had brought us together and that we have had almost 30 years of marriage to bring us to this point where my husband can care for me with so much love and compassion.

Email update to my team

Hi everyone—just wanted to say hi. Some of you have asked how I'm doing, so I thought I would let you know that I'm still in the game. God is so good and despite some minor complications, He showed me in small ways that He is watching over me. One example was in the middle of the night in the hospital. I was soooo tired and in pain and my roommate was so disruptive and I was reaching the end of my rope. My kids gave me an iPod for an early mother's day gift and so I put the buds in my ears with the only intention being to drown out hospital life. I randomly selected a worship compilation CD that I haven't listened to in years (Aaron loaded a bunch of stuff on it for me). A song came on that I had heard many times but had never really listened to the words. I listened to it 4 or 5 times in a row and cried. It touched my heart profoundly and I realized that no matter where I am, I am never alone and God is stronger than anything I am facing. The song is called "Stronger than the Storm".

I'm recuperating more slowly than I would like to but I have to remind myself that it hasn't been very long and it was a nasty surgery and I was still recovering from the first one. I'm looking forward to seeing the surgeon on Wed. to hopefully have my drain and stitches removed. I have a few weeks to recuperate and by then I should have the results of this last surgery and an appt. with the oncologist to start treatments.

Ron and I were talking today about how we could never put into words the feelings and emotions we are encountering as we go through this experience. If you've ever been in a situation similar to this, you know what I'm talking about. You people are the way God expresses His love to us. I never liked the expression "Jesus with skin on" because it sounded kind of gross, but it makes a lot of sense to me now. Thank you again for all the prayers and support and encouragement and flowers and food, etc.

Love,

Sherri (and Ron)

Eventually the drain was removed, and the dressings came off, but recovery was not complete. The surgery had damaged nerves in the back of my arm and the front of my upper arm, and I was also dealing with cording, which I found out meant scar tissue had adhered to muscle and/or blood vessels from my first incision through my underarm and all the way down to my elbow and eventually down to my wrist.

Email update to my team

Subject: How's Sherri doing?

I thought it's about time to let you know how I'm doing. I saw the dr. (surgeon) yesterday and had the rest of my bandages and stitches removed. She evaluated my arm movement and recommended physio to regain range of motion. A disappointing outcome of the last surgery was the residual nerve damage in the back of my shoulder and upper arm. Since surgery, I have had extreme nerve pain in these places and have had to take exorbitant amounts of drugs to cope with the pain. She is hoping that physio can help with this, too. She said this is a very rare complication with this surgery. Yay—I'm a special girl! But she says there is still a chance that the nerves can heal and the pain will lessen. Please pray for this healing. I am supposed to see the physiotherapist who specializes in this next week sometime.

I also want to tell you that I cherish your prayers for me and my family. We don't take this for granted in the least. Your encouraging emails are precious to me and keep me going just knowing people are remembering and praying. I've been rather down emotionally this past week with the pain of recovery, grieving the loss of control of my life, but even more so just the grim reality of what I have to face yet to get through to the other side of this nightmare. I really pray for joy in the journey but it's pretty hard some days. I hope you can take me being honest with you.

Thank you for praying for me.

Love,

Sherri

The next specialist I met with was a physiotherapist who specializes in working with breast cancer patients who are having trouble recovering from breast surgery. She also specializes in lymphedema, which I didn't have right away but have had some mild problems with since. What an amazing woman. She is so compassionate and knowledgeable. A great combination. And her services are covered by the provincial healthcare plan, so we don't need to worry about how to pay for it, which is also a really nice benefit.

EMAIL UPDATE TO MY TEAM

Subject: The Next Step

Hi everyone,

I'm glad the surgeries are behind me—and I want to thank you for your prayers and support through that stage. The physiotherapist told me last week that I have what is called "cording" in my upper arm, which means that scar tissue is holding some nerves and so I am massaging and stretching to loosen the scar tissue and get more mobility. It isn't a quick fix, but she's hopeful that I should be able to get my range of motion back and that the nerve pain will subside. I'm doing my physio exercises and I've already had a big improvement in my pain levels and so I thank you for praying for that. Don't stop praying for this though—I'm not quite there yet.

I also want to request prayer for tomorrow. I'm meeting with the oncologist at 10:45 to discuss the next step in the "C" journey—my treatment plan. I've read up on chemotherapy and have done some internet research, but until I actually meet with the boss who controls this part of my battle, I won't really know what I'm going to be facing. There are so many unknowns, and that makes me anxious. So I'm asking for prayer for peace again. God has answered those prayers in a very special way by giving me a calmness when I become overwhelmed and fearful, and I know it can only come from Him. It means that I am consciously choosing to trust Him with all of my hopes and my dreams and my future. That's not easy.

So thanks for praying...again.

I'll let you know how it turns out.

Love,

Sherri

Chapter Three
Oncology 101

The Next Step: Oncology

The next step on this road was to meet with the oncologist and set up a treatment plan. This was one of the toughest days, mentally and emotionally. After waiting for what seemed a really long time in the waiting area and then in the examining room, the doctor appeared in a fast and hurried state. He had my file in his hands but clearly had not even opened the cover. He examined me way too quickly and then informed me that the cancer I was dealing with had a high rate of recurrence, so I would need both chemo and radiation and did I have any questions, and if so, the nurse would answer them and then he was gone. Oh, my goodness. He hadn't taken the time to actually see me or hear me or get to know me. This was the man who literally had my life in his hands. He had said he didn't think I needed a port and thought I could have a PIC

IV (Peripherally Inserted Central Catheter) installed for the chemo treatments. After he left, I cried and told the nurse I needed to be able to trust the people who were taking care of me and it was so obvious he hadn't studied my file. I was concerned about my blood–clotting factor, and my IV history and I had thought I would need a port for the chemo treatments. I had pages of questions and after the doctor left the room. I felt so dismissed.

But the nurse was excellent, and she realized I was upset. She sat down and took the time to put me at ease and answer my questions. She told me I would absolutely be losing my hair, and explained the drugs that would be given during chemo. The chemo regimen is called 3x3—3 treatments of 3 drugs (Epirubicin, Fluorouracil, and Cyclophosphamide) and then 3 treatments of another (Taxotere). But I found out that before chemo could even start, I would need a battery of tests. It looked like chemo treatments would be weeks away yet, and I was so discouraged.

The saving grace for this doctor was that as we were leaving, he met us in the hallway and told us he had taken some time to read through my file and agreed that a port would be the best thing, and apologized for being in such a hurry with me. This was obviously without the nurse having said anything to him, because she was with us the entire time.

I think the hardest thing for me at this point was the painful realization that my dream of having cancer treatments done by the time the grandbabies were due was slipping away. I needed to realize it was an unrealistic expectation and I was going to have to let it go. This was really hard emotionally and so out of my control.

The nurse phoned us the very next day to let us know she had times and dates for the tests that needed to be done and they were set up for the very next week. She knew we wanted to get going as soon as possible and she was so encouraging.

Email update to my team

It's been a busy day. We met with the oncologist this morning. I don't know about you but I don't do well with having to wait. Ron says I was very fidgety. (Is that a word?) The appt. didn't go as we had hoped it would. It seems there are more things to take care of before chemo can begin. So I'm waiting for an appt. for a heart muscle strength test and an appt. to have a port (central line) put in (another day surgery at HSC). This needs to be done before I can start chemo, so it might be a few weeks yet. I also need to have a complete bone scan done and a CT of my chest and stomach to make sure there is no cancer lurking in those places. It's been a hard day emotionally and mentally. I really wanted to get started so I could be finished with treatments and healthy by the time my grandbabies arrive at the end of October, but that really can't happen now.

I also saw the physiotherapist this afternoon and she was pleased with the progress I was able to make in one week. I see her again next week. And then I went to see my chiropractor, who was finally able to adjust my lower back properly after trying to contort and invent new ways of adjusting it during 2 months of surgeries and recoveries. He also found that my collarbone was quite out of place and adjusted that, which made a huge difference right away in my arm's range of motion, which was good but painful.

I did have moments of peace in between. So thanks for praying for me today. Your emails are so encouraging. It makes such a difference to me and Ron and my kids to know that people care and are aware of what is happening here in our family. If you see my kids, give them a hug, k? They are being so strong but I know they worry.

Thanks.

Love,

Sherri

The Tests

The Bone Scan

Ron took me to the first test, which was the bone scan. It really was a non–event after the surgeries. One injection of radioactive dye at 11:00 in the morning and then we could leave the hospital and come back at 2:00. We thought shopping would take our minds off of the immediate, so we went to the mall and found some summer clothes for Ron. When we got back to the hospital, I had another injection and then was ushered into a room with the scanner. Before I laid down for the scan, which was supposed to take half an hour or more of lying perfectly still, I asked if I could use my iPod. The technicians told me it had never been done before but one of them said, "Why not? Nothing in the test is magnetic so it should be okay." So I was permitted to use my iPod and it was the best thing in the world. I went to my happy place and listened to my happy music and it went well. The only downside is the nagging fear of the results. Of course, I hope and pray and want the scan to come back with the result of no cancer in any of my bones, but the reality is still that it was found in my lymph nodes, so anything is possible. We left the hospital in good spirits knowing one test was done now and it had been an easy one.

The MUGA Scan

The next test was two days later. It is called a MUGA scan, and it tested the strength of my heart muscles to see if they could withstand the chemo drugs, which could potentially injure the heart muscles if they aren't strong enough. It was also radioactive. My sister, Laurie, was with me for this one. It also meant an injection and then waiting half an hour, which we spent in the waiting room discussing wigs and my potential lack of hair. It went by fast and soon I was back in the same scanner room with the same technicians and the discussion of using my iPod was a quick one. This test took a bit longer, but it was broken into five–to–eight–minute increments, and I could move around and reposition myself in between, which was good for my lower back.

After it was done, we needed to make a visit to the oncology department to meet with the nurse who was managing my case. She had information about the port installation, which was to take place on Monday. When we got in to see her, she unexpectedly had the results of the bone scan. It was really nice for Laurie to be there to hear the nurse inform us the results were all good. No cancer was found in any bones! We did a little dance and hugs all around—including the nurse. It was obvious she felt very happy to give me this news. It was so nice to have some good news for a change. I immediately called Ron and then each of my kids. I think all of them cried on the phone, as did I. What a relief!

Email update to my team

Subject: Better news

Hi. So this week has been crazy busy with tests and more tests. Today was the Muga scan, which sounds funny but is a heart muscle strength test. (To make sure that my heart can handle some of the chemo drugs that can cause heart damage) The scans this week have been quite uneventful and relatively painless. The one today was 2 injections of radioactive solutions half an hour apart, and in between I needed to go for a blood test—one of the 3–vial kinds and so I have 3 bandages on one arm today and feel a bit pin–cushiony. But I needed to go to the Vic. oncology today to speak to my nurse there after the scan was done and she had the results of my bone scan already. It's totally clear!!! What a huge relief. I needed some good news and wow I had no idea what a relief this would be. The tears flowed. Thank you, Jesus.

I also know already that I am going to have my port installed on Monday at 1:00 at the Health Sciences day surgery unit. I have 2 CT scans booked for next week Wed. and my first meeting with the radiology oncology dept. at St. Boniface after my scans that day.

And the date for my first chemo treatment is set for the Monday after, June 23rd.

Don't worry, I'll remind you of that date and time! The type of chemo regimen is called FEC in case you want to do some homework.

Good test results!

Thanks for prayer,

Love,

Sherri

The Port Installation

So the next step was the port installation, which I had researched and talked to others about. It seemed like a small procedure compared to what I had already gone through. This was scheduled for a Monday morning and I was told it would take about two hours from start to finish, and was a relatively non–invasive and simple thing to do. I was informed I probably wouldn't even need any pain medication. I fasted as I was advised to do, and after checking in at the day surgery unit at the Health Sciences Centre, I was given another lovely set of blue gowns (why are they always blue?) and matching slippers to change into. I was tucked into my bed by 11:00 and then proceeded to wait for my slated 1:00 appointment.

Because of my IV history, a "professional" IV team was supposed to come to start my IV so a sedative could be administered during the port installation procedure. A male wearing scrubs came to my bedside and informed me he was the IV specialist. He tried once, and failed. On the second try, I told him it didn't feel right and it was hurting me, but he tried to convince me it was a good IV and the procedure wasn't a long one, so any pain would be short–lived and it would be okay. I was given a hot towel to wrap my arm in to ease the pain and I resigned myself to it because I told myself that ironically this might be the last IV I would need to endure, because I was having a port installed. After waiting past my 1:00 time slot, we realized I had been somehow overlooked in the scheduling—someone came into my room and asked, "what is she waiting for?" And the other person told him, she's here for a port installation and he said, what, there's another one? So I was taken down to where the procedure would take place at about 2:00.

The first thing that took place here was the nurse checked my IV line, and when she started flushing it, I was in more pain and she informed me that this IV was no good. I couldn't believe the irony of the whole situation. I needed a port because it was too hard to start IVs and I needed an IV to have the port installed! I tried not to panic but I admit I was shaking and scrambling to remember some of the important Godly phrases or verses that had helped me through tough times in the past. The one that comes most readily is, "Thou wilt keep him in perfect peace whose mind is stayed on Thee," but with this comes the visual of my grade seven teacher, Mr. Hiebert, who taught us a song with this verse in it and I not only picture him, but hear his strong baritone voice as he directed the music class. Not necessarily a scene of tranquility. The other phrase that comes to me over and over is, "Be strong and courageous," and that's what I tried to be, but the tears spilled over as a second IV was attempted. This one was successful on the first try—I suggested that she be the designated professional IV person from now on!

Now I was ready for the port installation. Ron was told it would take approximately twenty minutes and was shown a waiting room. An hour later, he went to ask about me and was told there had been complications and it would be a while yet. After an hour–and–a–half, I was wheeled out of the room on a stretcher and Ron escorted me back to the day surgery unit.

The port installation procedure normally consists of the patient being given a sedative that puts them into a twilight zone—awake but not fully aware and having no memory of the procedure. Well, I was sedated but quite aware, and I remember the doctor instructing someone to keep giving me more drugs because I was too awake. I specifically remember one of the nurses in the room, because she panicked a bit when I told her both of my daughters were pregnant and one of them had been on the pill. She immediately wanted to know the brand of pill she had been on!

This young woman was my guardian angel during the procedure. I was lying on a table with my face and upper chest covered in sterile cloths. My head was turned and only one eye was visible. This nurse kept putting her face into view to talk to me and encourage me and reassure me. It really helped me get through it. The complication during this time was that because of my bad veins—again, ironically, the reason I needed the port—the doctor tried about five or six times to insert a catheter into veins in my chest and couldn't find one that could support the catheter. He finally resorted to cutting a slit in my neck and using my jugular vein to insert the catheter. This catheter is attached to the port, which was implanted into my chest muscle just above my right breast. Normally, the catheter would be sitting just below the collarbone. This catheter was threaded through the vein and into the superior vena cava. In my "twilight" state, I remember a lot of tugging and pressure and pulling.

When it was over, my angel nurse told me I would need pain medication and ice, because I would be very sore after what I had endured. So much for a simple procedure. When I got back to the day surgery unit, the nurses there were obviously expecting me and had heard about the complications. I was immediately given drugs and an ice pack. I went home with a very swollen neck and upper chest, but also down in the dumps about how something so simple could turn so complicated for me. Can't I do anything right? I know it was silly of me to think I could somehow blame myself for this, or even to think that I had any control over it. But I grew up being the "accident prone" girl in school. I used to have a closet full of casts as my souvenirs to prove it. In grade nine, I had two sets of stitches and two casts—all from separate incidents. I win.

Email update to my team

Subject: Sherri's mistake

Hi—I had a wake up call from the Lord today. I tried to do what I needed to do without reminding and asking people to pray for me. I thought I was going to be able to do this somewhat on my own. Big mistake. This port installation was supposed to be a walk in the park compared to what I've already experienced. Not so. I'll make this short, but the day included 3 IV attempts—by professionals—and one port installation that didn't go well. It is installed but it took multiple attempts and ended up using my neck as a portal for the catheter instead of the usual spot just under the collarbone. I am in much pain and maybe asking for prayer retroactively is okay, isn't it? I am quite swollen and not very happy, but glad that they finally got the port installed. I have a day off to recuperate now and then a full day on Wed. with CT scans starting at 9 in the morning, and several other appointments to fill the rest of the day. I'm still hoping and praying that chemo can start on Monday, the 23rd, as planned. Ron was again my pillow/pillar of strength and I praise the Lord for him.

Love,
Sherri

The CT Scan

Well, the port procedure had been accomplished, and I set out to heal so I could have my next test—the CT scan (Computed Axial Tomography). This scan would check all of my internal organs to see if the cancer had spread anywhere else in my body. This was scheduled to take place two days after the port was installed, but it was still so very swollen and I was quite concerned about it. I had been informed that a radioactive dye would be used for the scan and would need to be injected into the port. We called to discuss our concerns with the oncology nurse and she advised us to postpone the CT scan. She was concerned, too, and asked us to come in to get it checked for infection or rejection. We went back to the hospital and were treated very efficiently and so compassionately. After we were ushered into a treatment room, the oncology nurse, as well as an attending nurse, checked for any sign of infection and, seeing there was none, we were given the clearance to go home. I appreciated being treated as if this was important and not unnecessary. They were interested and a bit freaked out at my port installation story and my war wounds to show for it.

Hit in the Rear

The next big thing that happened also occurred the same week. On Thursday night, Ron's family was going out for supper to celebrate his parents' fifty–fifth wedding anniversary. I decided that even though I was still in quite a bit of pain, I would accompany Ron because this was important to him and the rest of the family. Driving to the restaurant, we were rear–ended by a young man who was apparently not focused on driving—he hit us as we were waiting for a red light to change. It was quite a jolt and my first reaction was not good. Too many years of working in Junior High conjured up some not–so–nice language. I could feel that my neck had been jarred, and I really didn't feel very excited about the prospect of dealing with whiplash on top of everything else my poor body was trying to cope with. Both of us had sore necks almost immediately, and knew we had been injured. After the pleasantries had been exchanged between the drivers, we headed for the restaurant. We would need to deal with the damage later, but we did worry about possibly needing to go vehicle shopping in the near future. Our CRV didn't seem to be very damaged, but we already had a claim on it for some hail damage a few weeks earlier, and this accident could make it a write off. We didn't want that to happen. Who has time to worry about a vehicle at this point in their story?

Not Another One

During the past two months, we had been very aware that close friends of ours are also walking through the cancer scare. My girlfriend, who is two years younger than I am, had a swollen spot on her neck and went to get it checked out. From the first doctor she saw in Emergency, she was told cancer was the most likely diagnosis, but that it couldn't be confirmed without tests. She came over one morning after her tests, and even though she didn't have her results yet, we commiserated because we both knew the tone and expressions used by doctors who know but just can't tell you yet. We know now that she was dealing with Lymphoma.

Her husband has been an "accountability brother" for my husband for quite a few years, and it's absolutely awesome that these two have such a strong relationship and were able to walk through this valley together and support each other. I'm sure they never thought this would be what they were building each other up for all of these years. Both of us cancer chicks are so blessed to have these guys in our lives.

Chapter Four
Chemotherapy

Start of Chemo

June 23, 2008

The most important thing I did before we left for the hospital for my first treatment was to enlist the aid of my prayer support team. I sent them all an email to remind them to pray for me, and for us. It's very important to make sure the people you are counting on for support and encouragement are aware of what is happening.

Email to my team

Subject: Chemo is starting

Hi everyone,

I thought I would send a reminder on Sunday for people to pray for me on Monday when I will be going for my first chemo treatment at 10:00 a.m., but as the weekend looms before me, I'm realizing that I need prayer now. I'm so glad to be starting the treatments, because that means I'll be done someday soon. But the other part of me is so scared and worried. I've had so many complications in the past week and I'm feeling quite down about it all. The port site and neck are still quite sore and swollen but as a complication, the lymph glands in the other original incision site are swollen too, as well as some further cording and lymphedema starting in the left arm. I need prayer for chemo to go well on Monday but also for the other problems I mentioned. The plan is to freeze the port site so it can be used on Monday. I would really like to be able to relax and enjoy this weekend with my family at the lake without worrying about chemo on Monday, so pray for some of that supernatural peace that only God can give. I need to be able to give my burdens to Him and know that He loves me and is taking care of me. He is an amazing God and I know without a doubt that He has been with me, as I've survived many things in the past 2 months that I could never imagine having gotten through on my own. Please also don't forget to pray for Ron and my kids and kids–in–law. This is a scary journey for everybody involved.

Thank you for respecting my wishes about not forwarding my emails on to other people without asking me first. It's really important to me to know that this group of email supporters are safe so I can be personal and honest about my struggles. I don't mind you sharing my requests for prayer with others—just don't send my emails on. Thanks.

Love,

Sherri

I have to say I was quite anxious about my first appointment for chemo. I've told you before that I'm not a saint. I was greeted by a very nice nurse at the treatment centre door and she informed me that I would be having my first treatment in a private room. She was assigned to take care of me—from answering any questions before we started, to actually administering the drugs, watching me like a hawk, and serving me snacks. She was absolutely awesome and my fears vanished—well, almost completely—as she explained everything that would happen even before it happened. I sure wished I could have taken her home to continue taking care of me. The entire treatment lasted four–and–a–half hours—a bit longer than usual, because I developed a headache and was given an extra bag of saline to flush my system. And the port worked! What a relief. That was probably causing most of my anxiety. I was given a patch of something to freeze the site when we first arrived. It wasn't completely frozen after half an hour, but my helpful nurse seemed to be eager to start and so were we. It hurt a bit, mostly from the pressure of poking the needle into the port. But it worked. Hallelujah.

The first drug, Epirubicin (Ellence), was actually three huge syringes of red fluid, and I was warned I would be peeing pink for a while. She told me this drug would be the main culprit of my impending hair loss. The nurse pulled up a stool and let me know she would be spending some quality time with me, as she needed to inject each syringe very slowly into my IV line. The process for this drug administration probably took about half an hour, but the time passed really quickly as we became acquainted. We compared the ages of our children, swapped work stories, and discussed life prior to cancer.

My line was flushed and the second drug, Fluorouracil (5FU), was administered the same way, except it was only one small syringe full of clear liquid. I was given more saline and I soon realized I would need to go for walks to the washroom quite frequently with this amount of fluid, combined with the cups of water and apple juice I was encouraged to drink. It was great to have Ron there so he could follow behind me, guiding my friend, Mr. IV Pole.

The third drug, Cyclophosphamide (Cytoxan), was an IV drip—just a bag hung up on the pole—and I didn't even notice it except for the headache I told you about. A kind of funny thing happened before the headache…my nose became super sensitive and it felt like I was sniffing very strong alcohol. It was stinging up into my forehead and then the headache came on. At this point, we really didn't know if the headache could be whiplash–related from our recent accident, because we still hadn't had the opportunity to get that checked out. The nurse said it could be anxiety–related or it could be a reaction to one of the chemo drugs. She flushed another bag of saline through my IV just to see if that might help the headache, and then we were on our way home. I kept thinking, this is all? I was just waiting for the nausea and yuckiness to hit, but it didn't. Not right away, anyway…

Email update to my team

Subject: Thank you for your chemo prayers

Thank you, Thank you, Thank you.

I'm not sure what to tell you except that I couldn't help but smile during the chemo treatment today. I felt "held", which is an awesome feeling to have—held by God in the palm of His hand, held by my awesomest husband and best kids in the world, held by my friends and family.

The answers to prayer that I experienced today were:

- the port worked! I was quite concerned about this, because of the difficulty in installing it. When the nurse administered the chemo drugs through the IV connected to the port, I didn't feel a thing. What a relief!
- so far no actual throwing up. My stomach is unsettled, but the good drugs are doing their job.
- really great nursing staff in the oncology dept.

Thank you so much for keeping me (us) in your prayers! And now for the next few days, could you please pray for everything to settle down? I am dealing with a chemo headache and achy muscles right now and some prayer would be appreciated. Apparently tomorrow is supposed to be the worst of it.

Also, please don't forget to thank God for His answers.

Love,

Sherri (and Ron)

The next forty–eight hours are a bit of a blur due to the headache. After the drug, Epirubicin, I was commanded—yes, commanded—to drink liquids to flush out my system if I didn't want permanent damage to my kidneys and bladder. I was told to drink at least four litres a day and not to stop for the night. Of course, the side effect of this is having to go to the bathroom every half–hour. Because of the steroids, I couldn't really sleep anyway, so getting up to drink and pee during the night wasn't a big problem. You need to take the steroids (Kytril—six pills in total) to keep the nausea and vomiting at bay, but I was glad to be finished taking them after the second day because I felt more like myself and could sleep much better.

Some other side effects I experienced:

- A red, flushed face and upper chest. I called the oncology nurse and she thought it might be sunburn from driving home from the hospital. It was a hot, sunny day and she thought I might have burned through the car window. This didn't sound logical to me but I was too sick to care much and just lived with it. I put some aloe vera cream on it, but it didn't bother me at all.
- A red patch on my affected breast, also swollen and uncomfortable. The oncologist said it was not anything to be concerned about. The physiotherapist I have been seeing for my range of motion and lymphedema for my affected arm told me it was swollen because of the excess fluids I was consuming and it was pooling in my incision site. She massaged it so the fluids could drain, and it felt much better.
- Queasy stomach. I had the drugs to combat this, but didn't use them enough the first time. I'm not sure why. I think it was a combination of hav-

ing so many drugs in my system already and not wanting to take anything else and also just feeling too sick to think clearly. I used them more for the next treatment and it made a difference.

- Headache and more headache. It started during the last part of the chemo treatment and let up occasionally, but it was kind of migraine–like. Light hurt my eyes, and my head throbbed at my temples and the back of my head. Ron called the oncology nurse for advice about it and she suggested trying to get me to eat more. This actually helped, even though it was quite hard to do on a queasy stomach.
- Taste distortions. After two days, most food had very little taste to it and it was hard to eat. Some food tasted great for the first three or four bites and then the metallic aftertaste would come and spoil it. This didn't last very long. Most food taste was quite normal after a week and it was manageable.
- Mouth sores and cracking of my lips. I was given a popsicle to eat while I was being given the drug that causes mouth sores, so I thought I wouldn't get this side effect. Two days after my treatment, I realized my mouth was very dry and my tongue felt coated and yucky. I also had really sensitive gums. I bought toothpaste for sensitive teeth and a very soft toothbrush. My throat also began to get sore so I started gargling with salt water. I had some special mouthwash from the dentist. None of this really seemed to make a difference. I called a woman who had battled breast cancer a few years ago and asked her for help. She advised me

to try a natural product—Oil of Oregano drops—from a health food store. I tried it and it worked quickly. It tastes awful, so I put three drops in about a quarter–cup of milk and gargled twice a day, and after two days, my mouth and throat were pretty much back to normal. I even ate pizza by the end of my second week after chemo! For my cracked lips, the pharmacist recommended a suave called Carmex, which was very soothing and also worked fast to fix the problem.

- Fatigue. This is a side effect that needs to be talked about more. I think this is just your body telling you to take it easy and let the drugs do their job. They are supposed to kill off the white blood cells, so while they're doing that, you need to help them by resting and not trying so hard to do what you think you need to be doing. This was frustrating for me. I was used to working full time or, this past year, going to school and studying, reading and doing assignments more than full time, so this whole business of napping in the afternoons or dropping off to sleep every time we got into a vehicle felt like a real waste of time. But I tried to remember that if this was what I needed to do to recover, it made sense to give myself permission to rest and take care of myself and not worry about it. It's all part of the fight. It's also about losing control and letting others take care of you. This was also very hard for me. I would much rather be the one caring for someone else than be the recipient of others taking care of me. I needed to learn how to ask for help and appreciate it, instead of just coping and not asking or

> feeling bad for asking. It's also kind of cool when my husband and kids can recognize my fatigue levels and send me to bed. I don't want to miss out on anything, so it's hard to go for a rest, but it's easier when they see me zoning out and my eyes glazing over and order me to go for a nap!

Email update to my team

Subject: Chemo round 1 update

Hi Everyone,

Well, I thought I should let you know that I'm up and about again. Thank you for your prayers. There were times this past week when I thought about how many people were praying for me and it gave me the strength I needed. It wasn't a walk in the park. The terrible nausea and other nasty stuff never truly surfaced, but the drug (steroid) you have to take to counteract that produced a massive headache that hung around way too long. I'm hoping this can be tweaked for the next round. So I'm definitely on the upswing—eating better, sleeping better and feeling better.

Days 7–14 of this cycle are my low blood–count days and I'm supposed to avoid any sick germs, so if you're planning to visit, you'll see the hand disinfectant at the front door. Please use it. Any infection now could land me in the hospital, apparently. But that doesn't mean you should stay away. Except for fatigue right now, I'm feeling better than I have in a long time, so I would love to see you. Not all at the same time though! Unfortunately, this means no shopping, no movies , and no restaurants for the next week.

Ron is officially going back to work starting tomorrow, so some daytime company would be appreciated.

Have a great holiday today.

God is good,

Love,

Sherri

Where Did It Go?—My Hair Loss

Okay, this was a bit freaky. I knew this was coming and inevitable, but all the books say it happens about three weeks after the first treatment. I thought I had at least another week to go, but we were at the lake on a Sunday morning exactly two weeks after my treatment when I woke up and felt loose hairs on my face. I pulled them off and it hit me—I'm losing my hair! I had packed the hair clippers (and baseball cap) just in case, but really didn't expect this to happen yet. I lay in bed and did a tug test just for kicks. Out it came. I tried again, and yup…I was losing my hair. I thought it would be scarier or more traumatic, but I felt completely calm. My thinking was that it was good to get this milestone over with instead of living in dread and wondering when it was going to happen. It grossed me out to think of hair dropping into my food or onto my shoulders, so I wanted it shaved immediately.

My daughter Lindsay and her husband were still sleeping in the other room in the camper, and my husband had gone for an early morning fishing trip. I tiptoed into the adjoining room and woke Lindsay up. I told her what was happening and she wanted proof, so I did another tug and then she believed me. She teared up and I think was more affected by this than I was. It might have been her pregnancy hormones, but she cried more than I did.

Ron got back from fishing and asked what was going on. I told him he would need to shave my head. He couldn't believe it either and suggested I go shower first, and then we would see if I needed to be shaved. I didn't say anything. I reached up to my head with both of my hands and, without any effort, tugged two tufts of hair free and held them out to him. The shock on his face made me and Lindsay burst out laughing. It was a great stress reliever. He said, "Okay, I believe you. I'll go get the clippers." He shaved my head in the tiny bathroom of the camper while my cheering section watched from the front room.

After we were done, we ate breakfast and then I put on my baseball cap and we went to check out a show–and–shine car show in town. I wandered from car to car with Lindsay and we walked at about the same pace, with her pregnancy, my condition, and our mutual disinterest in seeing the cars! We ended up finding some hot chocolate and sharing a cinnamon bun as we waited for Geoff and Ron to take their time. I felt energized about having this hair loss milestone over with, and almost empowered at my lack of drama or stress about it all. It was great to have Lindsay (and Geoff) there for moral support.

Email update to my team

Subject: Another milestone

Hi everybody,

I just wanted to let you know that I am doing really well. I actually feel better physically than I have for probably 3 months—since before the first surgery. Other than a queasy stomach occasionally, very little appetite and frustrating fatigue, that's about it right now. I'm hoping that if I can bounce back after my first treatment, I can do it again for the second round and the third and...

My big milestone today was waking up with loose hair on my face and then realizing, Oh, my goodness, this is it. It's way too early though, the books say 3 to 4 weeks after the first treatment and it's only been 2 for me. But who's kidding, I'm not really doing anything by the books, am I? I did a little tug test lying there in bed and yup, it's coming out. Ron had the job of shaving my head while Geoff and Lindsay cheered us on in the next room. We were at the lake and I had packed the clippers just in case. So that's it then. I don't need to live in dread of this day coming anymore. I have my baseball cap, a few other head coverings, and a wig (a whole other neat story—a total God experience—coming through for us because we have no medical coverage for this adventure). It's all good. Thank you so much for your continued support and your very encouraging and uplifting emails. I cherish them and love you all so much for it.

Now let me know how I can pray for you.

Love,

Sherri

Some things "they" don't tell you about hair loss. Warning—some of this might be too much information or "over–share."

First of all, I became itchy and a bit sore in my privates, and then realized that every time I wiped, more and more pubic hair was falling out. This started about two days before the hair on my head fell out. I was told by a friend to watch the shower drain because it can get plugged by the hair loss. I put a piece of toilet paper over the drain and it caught most of the hair. Also, another person told me her head hurt like she had bumped it on something just before her hair came out, and I had the same experience. Actually, I could tell which part of my head would be losing hair by where it hurt. It's not a constant ache—just where you touch, it is sensitive.

Also, it's not a magical one–time deal when you lose your hair. Even after I shaved my head, I had bristles to deal with. Three weeks after my treatment, I had mangy patches of baldness mixed with bristles. And the bristles I still had were very annoying. My head hurt like I had tiny needles poking into it whenever I lay down or rested my head. I was waiting for the straggly bristles to fall out, but it wasn't happening, so I finally asked my husband to shave me bald just to get rid of them. We were advised not to do this because of risk of nicking the skin and infection, but I didn't know what else to do. They weren't going anywhere on their own. I shed a few tears during this shaving process because now I was totally bald. It felt really weird. But it was a relief to have this taken care of and it was also another intimate time with my husband. I felt very loved as he painstakingly and very gently shaved my head in our small bathroom. The plus side to this is that I didn't need to shave my legs or underarms, which was an unexpected side benefit during the summer months.

Some things I did after my chemo treatment surprised me. I felt well enough to go for bike rides at the lake, long walks and even some shopping. I didn't know how my body would react and I wasn't sure what to expect, so having time in between treatments when I felt really good was such a blessing. I can't imagine trying to hold down a job while taking treatments, but I felt well enough to enjoy life about five days after each treatment.

My Wonderful Wig Story

After my first treatment, I knew the countdown was on for losing my hair. I was getting anxious about not having any head coverings or even a wig. I was waiting for someone to have the time to go with me and it seemed like everyone was too busy. After I felt well enough, I finally made an appointment to visit a woman who runs a wig shop in our vicinity. She came highly recommended and is mentioned on the provincial CancerCare website, so I thought it seemed like a good place to start looking. I was prepared to drive myself, but I called my daughter Jessica and she was excited to go with me that afternoon. Just as we were about to leave, my husband came home from work and asked if he could tag along. So I ended up not going by myself, which was great. I felt blessed that they would want to come with me. The shop was in a house and it was cozy. She even had a big old rabbit hopping around. We sat down to wait for the wig lady and both Jessie and I saw a wig that looked just like my original hair sitting there on a shelf. It was even the same hair color I have had for years—fresh from the hairdresser. The price tag was high, and I knew it was out of my range. We have no medical insurance, so this would need to come straight out of our own pockets. I concentrated on a few head coverings I thought would suffice and decided I wouldn't get a wig.

The wig shop owner came to help us and asked if there was any wig I wanted to try on. I told her my financial situation and said I couldn't afford one. She asked if there was any wig I would try if I could afford one. I showed her the one we had seen and she insisted I try it on. It was incredible. It looked like me. Even Jessie said the back looked just like me. This compassionate lady told us she wasn't running this business just to make money, and she chose a few women each year who she wanted to bless and help to make the cancer journey just a bit easier. So she told us she wanted to reduce the price of the wig to make it affordable, and the rest would be her donation to CancerCare. She also gave me reductions on the head coverings I found, and even gave me a two–for–one deal. I was so humbled by this woman's generosity, and felt like I had been touched by an angel when we walked out of there. She even threw three pens into the leopard print bag of goodies. She gave me a huge hug and words of encouragement when we left. This was such an answer to prayer, and my anxiety about losing my hair was pretty much over because it was taken care of now.

I had another encouraging experience before I lost my hair. We had been looking for baby gifts for our daughters, and we found the perfect play–yards at Sears. I went with my husband to pick them up. The salesclerk who helped us asked me a few questions and wanted to know if the recipient of these play–yards was having twins. I told her I was going to have two grandbabies very close together and I also mentioned I was being very careful about germs because of having had a chemo treatment. She informed me that her sister–in–law had just finished her treatments for breast cancer and had left on a vacation to Ireland with her husband to celebrate. She told me there was life after breast cancer treatment and gave me a hug and wished me all the best. It wasn't awkward at all and I felt uplifted by the encouragement this complete stranger gave me. I hope after this is over I can be an encouragement like that to someone else.

Email update to my team

Subject: CT Scan—prayer requested

Hi everyone,

Just want to ask for prayer for tomorrow. I know a CT scan is peanuts compared to everything else but I'm feeling anxious about it. I know that I'll need to fast for 4 hours before it and then I'll need to drink some vile substance, and I'm not sure how that's going to go on an already queasy stomach. I also know that a radioactive substance will be injected into my port and I know that's supposed to be a relatively easy thing to do but I don't do things the easy way. So yes, I'm anxious. I'm also really trying to leave the results of this scan in God's hands because ultimately I have no control over it, but it's hard. I also really have no desire to set foot in a medical building again. I've been feeling so good this past week that I have times when I forget that I'm in cancer treatment. Going back to the hospital reminds me all over again and is also a wakeup call that my 2nd treatment is next week and I'm not looking forward to it. I know, one day at a time.

So I'm asking for prayer again—for peace and strength and calm. Please pray for things to go smoothly tomorrow and that the results will be clear with no other cancer found anywhere in my body. The scan is scheduled for noon.

Thanks,

I'll let you know how it goes.

Love,

Sherri

After my first treatment, I was given an appointment for the CT scan I had originally postponed. Now that my port was working, I could have it done. This took place a week after my chemo treatment, and I felt up to getting it out of the way. It seemed like just a formality, but as the date loomed closer, I became more and more anxious. "What if...the cancer has spread and I've just been complacent about the seriousness of it all? What if...I have way more cancer than anybody has predicted or been aware of? How can I possibly handle bad news like that?"

So I went into this CT scan fearing the worst but hoping for the best. They informed me I would need to drink something before the scan, but they neglected to tell me it would be three cups full of a vile concoction they call "peach juice", which I would need to drink on an empty stomach as I had been fasting since the night before. It will be a long time before I will be able to drink anything labelled peach juice again. The first cup wasn't too bad, and I gulped it down as quickly as possible. The second cup was to be downed half an hour after the first. By that time, it was warm and nastier than ever. I had a really rough time with this one and had to fight retching it back up. I was told I would be given a third cup just before the actual scan. I waited an hour before I was finally called in for the scan and yes, I was handed the third cup of peach juice at the door of the scan room. I drank it as fast as I could and it stayed down, thankfully.

Now came the tough part…the technician started looking for a vein to put in the IV so she could inject the radioactive dye. I told her I thought she would be using my port and she informed me that a port couldn't be used for this because it was a pressurized injection and it would blow my port. I was quite upset about this, because the reason we postponed the CT scan was because my port site was too sore to be used at the time of my original appointment! She made a call to the oncology department to talk to the nurse there and let her know she could not use my port. The oncology nurse warned her she would probably have a great deal of trouble putting in an IV, and advised her to call an IV expert. So she did call for the "PIC nurse" who, she told me, was the expert IV person, but she said she had lots of experience in this, so she would just check for a vein and if she didn't think she could do it, she would wait for the expert. Well, by that time I was in tears and she knew how upset I was. I kept thinking, again, that there is no way I could let anybody else know about this, so people will think everything is going okay. I can't get up and run to the waiting room to let Ron know. This is just between me and God again. So I gave it over to Him as I lay there in my beautiful blue gown, again, and let Him have His way. The technician wrapped my arm in a warm towel, which was actually quite soothing, and talked me through what she was doing. She found a vein she thought she could use and miraculously got it in on the very first try and we were set to go. After this, the actual scan was uneventful and was over quickly. She told me her name so that if I needed another scan in the future, I could ask for her, because I knew she could put in the IV successfully. It was a relief to get the scan over with, but now the waiting for the results would begin and that is an emotional battle that can't be adequately described…

Email update to my team

Subject: I'm back

Thank you so much for praying and for letting me know that you would be praying. The things they don't tell you… The three cups of peach juice were bad and I just told myself—be strong and courageous— as I was trying to drink it. I knew there had to be something I was justified in being anxious about and it wasn't revealed to me until I was already in my lovely blue gown and in the scanner room with the technician. She informed me that she couldn't use my port (which had been frozen for 2 hours already waiting for the IV injection) and would need to start an IV!!! The reason I had the port installed was to avoid this! Oh, the irony. My immediate reaction was to ask if I could go tell Ron in the waiting room so he could pray for me but I realized this was again, one of those times when I was on my own—me and Jesus (and everybody else who was praying). Phone calls were made and the special IV nurse was called in but before she arrived, this technician had heard my concerns and, after wrapping my arm in a hot towel, she was able to insert the IV successfully on her very first try! What a relief. I knew my Jesus had heard my silent cries for help and came to my rescue. The scan itself was no trouble at all. So we're home now and it's done PTL. Now I have 4 days of nothing medical. Yeah!

Love,

Sherri

I now had two glorious weeks without any medical appointments to worry about, until my next blood test to determine if my blood counts were sufficient to go ahead with my second treatment...except for the results of my CT scan looming over my head. I tried so hard to just enjoy life without worrying about it and I did manage to do that.

EMAIL UPDATE TO MY TEAM

Subject: Round 2

Hi everybody,

What a great weekend at the lake! Lots of rain and wind and no hydro for all of Sat. night and yet it was peaceful and relaxing. We spent time with friends and family and also had lots of time by ourselves. We went on a great bike ride this morning and I almost feel ready to go for chemo round 2. These past 2 weeks have been so good for me and it's hard to know that I'm going to be sick again. But I'm praying, and hope you will too, that I can bounce back again enough to enjoy some time before round 3. I realize that this is all for my own good and to make sure that the cancer is gone from my body.

So I'm emailing to ask for prayer for tomorrow—blood test (at 9) to see if I can have round 2 and to meet with my oncologist (at 11) to get test results (hopefully the CT scan results as well as the blood test) and to discuss my chemo side effects and see if we can tweak the dosages so I won't have to deal with the headache this time around. He was soooo busy last time I saw him, I just wasn't very impressed. I would really like to walk out of there tomorrow with a better feeling of mutual trust and respect.

If the blood counts are good, then I'll be set to go for Round 2 on Wed. at 11.

If you're reading this before you go to bed tonight, could you please pray that I can relax enough to have a good sleep?

Also pray for peace and strength for tomorrow as well as on Wed. (if I can have my next chemo— pray that I can) and especially for the side effects to be minimal and that I can bounce back again.

Thanks again for your support and prayer.

Love,

Sherri

I feel like now that the first chemo treatment and recovery is over, talking about the second treatment seems redundant. There are no new revelations—just getting through the first five days, and then life resumes as a new kind of normal. I'm getting used to being bald, even though I still spook myself when I see my reflection in the mirror or a window. It's kind of cool that I can actually forget I'm bald. That means I'm comfortable with it but also that the people in my life have become comfortable with it, too. I've had a few awkward experiences though—like when we stopped at the gas station on the way to the lake and I was waiting in line to use the women's washroom. There was an older lady behind me and I could see her reflection in the bathroom mirror. I don't think she realized I could see her. The first look on her face said she was asking herself if I was indeed a woman and whether I should be in this line. I was wearing a baseball cap and I realized later that I had forgotten to put in my earrings! The second look said, "I wonder if she has cancer...?" And then she just kept looking and I don't really know what she was thinking. But it was awkward and I cried afterward when I told Ron. It's not like I had a say in this or that going bald was my choice. So many things are out of my control and one of them is the reactions of other people.

Another awkward time was when my sister Val's daughter, who was two years–old, pointed at me and said, "Funny hair." A short time later, she climbed onto the lawn swing beside me and tried to pull off my baseball cap. She asked to see my hair. I told her there is no hair there to see and I chose to keep my cap on. I didn't want to be the reason she would have nightmares or require therapy when she is older.

There have been other times when people chose to take a

second and third look and when I looked at them, they turned away. It hurts. Where are all of the other chemo patients who can relate? It would be so cool if a stranger would say something like, "Hey, I know what you're going through and it's going to be okay." But I haven't seen any other woman at Falcon Lake who is bald and out in public. Do all other chemo patients stay at home where it is safe? I just can't live my life that way. For me, that's not living life—that's just coping. It's also not fair that it's okay for guys to be bald but not for a woman! Did you ever notice how many guys choose to be bald? They shave their entire head and it's just fine—society accepts this as normal. Not fair.

Well, I went for my blood test for chemo round two and got the results of my CT scan. This is the email I sent to my email support team…

EMAIL UPDATE TO MY TEAM

Subject: Pre–Chemo Round 2

It's a go for tomorrow. My blood test was amazing (except for the port not working right but it was okay). A normal white blood count is between 4 and 11 and mine came back at 8.8, which apparently is very, very good. We discussed the chemo cocktail for tomorrow and the steroid we suspect is giving me the headaches is too important for controlling the nausea and vomiting to take out of the mix, so I'm going to try it again. I was armed with some suggestions for pain meds and for getting more nutrients into my system to counteract the headache.

I also want to share with you that my CT scan results came back and I'm very happy to announce that everything came back clear!!!! A very small nodule (2mm) was found in the lining of my right lung, but the dr. assured me that he doesn't think it is cancer related at all, but will be keeping an eye on it in the future. I also have some fibroid cysts in my uterus, which I will need to have an ultrasound for just to check them out, but he also says this is very common and not malignant. So I am (we are) breathing a huge sigh of relief. I have to confess that even with your prayers, my sleep was not good last night because of worrying about these results. It was the last remaining piece of my prognosis puzzle and a pretty significant one. I feel like I can look forward to the future with so much more hope and optimism with these results.

Thanks again for keeping me in your prayers and please continue for this week with chemo and recovery.

Love you all and appreciate you so much,

Sherri

Email update to my team

Subject: Chemo Round 2

Well, I have to say that round 2 has definitely been better so far than the first one. I think we worked out some kinks and my body is just handling it better. I have felt pretty good today, except for that same "sunburn" I dealt with the first time. I was told to come in to get it checked out if it happened again this time, and it did. So we went back to the hospital this afternoon and were told it was a mild reaction to one of the drugs, and to keep a close eye on it. But it cleared up the first time, so I assume it will again once the drugs are flushed from my body. I have been dealing with a minor headache all day and I'm praying it doesn't get worse overnight. So far it's been quite manageable.

Thanks again for all of your prayers. The actual chemo session went well. The port worked 100% and I had a great discussion with the nurse who was administering my drugs about Human Resource Management and how to retain and manage young employees! We were done in 3 hours this time. Both Ron and I were much less anxious just knowing what to expect and both of us expressed how much peace we felt. God is so good.

My third day was the hardest one as far as side effects go (the first time), so I'm praying it will go well tomorrow and I will recover without complications and be able to enjoy another 2 weeks of summer with friends and family after this. Yesterday morning I kept thinking that by the afternoon, I would only have 4 more rounds of chemo left to go and that actually sounds doable!

Thanks again for your prayers and encouragement.

Love,

Sherri

Chapter Five

More Than Enough

Through all of this, I've had very distinct God moments. I'm going to include an email I sent in the wee hours of the morning a few weeks ago, because I think it's fresher and more real when it's the original.

Email to my team

Subject: Midnight Rant

Hi. I know this is the middle of the night and I don't normally do this...but God prompted me to get out of bed and write this. It's His fault—complain to Him. Warning—this is a spiritual rant.

This morning was one of those God mornings when "coincidences" happened and I know there is no other explanation than God wanting to give me a message and apparently share it with you...

It started with Lindsay's blog. I read it and a song popped into my head, "Enough"—a worship song that talks about God being more than enough to supply every need. My family can attest to the fact that I always have random songs going through my head at any given moment, so this isn't a new phenomenon, but apparently it's really annoying when it spills out. But the point is that this was the song that was in my head. I went to the living room and picked up my devotional book and opened it to where the bookmark was from the last time I read it, and the title of the devotional for today was "More than Enough." I read it and it was exactly what I needed. I knew in my heart that God had orchestrated this and wanted to give me the message that no matter what I am going through, He is more than enough to walk through it with me and carry me when I need to be carried. He is the one who supplies me with the strength and hope and peace and joy I need to get through this cancer valley.

So I wanted to write you to encourage you in whatever you are going through in your lives. I repeat I'm not a saint. I'm a normal person trying to navigate life just like you. But if you're trying to do life on your own—whether you've had a personal relationship with Jesus Christ at some point and "lost" Him in the busyness of life, or chosen to put your relationship on hold…or have never had that personal relationship with Him ever…I just can't imagine trying to get through this without Him. He has shown me He is aware of what I'm dealing with in many precious ways that can only be explained as supernatural. His spirit is speaking to me and opening my eyes to be aware of the messages He is giving me. It's so awesome. I also want to tell you I'm not working right now—just going through treatments and trying to beat this. But I have time to read emails, talk to you (personally, not on the phone, please), or come on over. I have time to listen, and to pray for you. Let me know how I can pray for you.

K, I better try to get some sleep. I think that's all. I'm recovering well from my second chemo—not quite 100% but working on it. ;)

Thanks for listening…

Love,

Sherri

I had an amazing number of replies to this email. I had no idea so many people under my own nose were dealing with tough stuff going on in their lives. Now I had given them permission to share their burdens with me.

One of these people was a woman from my church who has been a constant encourager for me in the past few months and a special woman in my eyes. She called me up one day and asked me what I was hungry for, because she wanted to bring me lunch. She picked up some sub sandwiches and came over to share them with me. It was really cool for her to do that. As we ate, she told me what was going on in her life, and she's been going through some pretty nasty stuff, too—not cancer related at all, but that doesn't make it any easier to deal with. So we prayed together and then she left, and I felt like maybe I wasn't done with my life. I could still help others carry their burdens and make their loads a bit lighter and God would honour that. If others were helping me carry my load, I had room to carry some of theirs. It just made sense to me. This woman and all of the others who emailed responses to my middle of the night rant affirmed me in this. I was happy I had listened and obeyed God's prompting.

These song lyrics were dancing in my head that morning…

Enough

Written by Chris Tomlin/Louie Giglis

You are my supply
My breath of life
Still more awesome than I know.
You are my reward
Worth living for
Still more awesome than I know.

And all of you
Is more than enough for
All of me
For every thirst and every need
You satisfy me with your love
And all I have in you is more than enough

More Than Enough

You're my sacrifice
Of greatest price
Still more awesome than I know.
You're my coming King
You're my everything
Still more awesome than I know.

And all of you
Is more than enough for
All of me
For every thirst and every need
You satisfy me with your love
And all I have in you is more than enough
You are more than enough.

More than all I want
More than all I need
You are more than enough for me.
More than all I know
More than all I can see
You are more than enough for me.

All of you
Is more than enough for
All of me
For every thirst and every need
You satisfy me with your love
And all I have in you. (Oh Yeah)
And all I have in you. (Jesus)
And all I have in you is more than enough.[1]

My Great Escape

Our trailer at the lake became my haven. We went out there as often as possible and enjoyed times by ourselves and with our family and friends, in between chemo treatments during the summer of 2008 and beyond. Since then, God has blessed us with a seasonal site at the same campground every summer. It is a place of healing for me as we take walks and bike rides, go fishing and watch the sunset on the water. I realized that summer that God isn't only in a church building on a Sunday morning. We weren't attending church regularly during that summer, because I was too afraid of the germ contact, but also because I felt so fragile emotionally and didn't want to make a scene in public. I found God as I sat on a bench at the beach and I talked to Him there as I looked out over the water. He isn't a God who wants to be stuck in a box. He is the God of the universe and He delights in His children appreciating His marvellous creations.

Two experiences at the trailer that summer were very meaningful to me and I thought were significant enough to share.

The first one took place when I spent a few days there with Laurie. I was in the middle of my chemo treatments, and she was recovering from surgery, so we were quite the sight shuffling along on our many walks. We shared our hearts during our time together, and one of our heart–to–heart conversations took place in a restaurant at the lake. She told me she wasn't ready to give me up, and that she wasn't even going to think about the possibility of me dying until the time came that she would need to. I felt sick to my stomach. Maybe a chemo reaction, or the restaurant food, but I actually had a physical reaction to what she was saying. I shared with her that I needed for her to release me. I asked her to give God the freedom to do His work in my life. I wasn't giving up and was still determined to fight my fight, but with the knowledge that

I was in God's hands and there are no guarantees in life. I felt like I needed to be able to go through the recommended treatments without the pressure of having to "make it" for other people. We shed tears and hugged a lot that weekend. It was special and I felt like a load had been lifted.

The second experience was my own little planned escape. Ron didn't like the idea of me spending time at the lake by myself, but it was something I really wanted to do. I wanted some uninterrupted "me" time. I wanted to go for walks and lie in the hammock and spend time talking to God and writing down my thoughts. It was time for me to wrestle through some things with God and find peace with my Maker. It was after my second treatment and just before my third. I wrote down my thoughts as they came to me during those few days so I could process them better. When I get them down on paper, I feel I don't have to hold them in my head anymore. When I can see my thoughts in actual words, it helps me to realize how ridiculous they are, or, on the other hand, how profound my thoughts are sometimes (in my opinion, of course). I also feel like God can speak to me when I verbalize my thoughts, either by saying them to Him or by writing them down.

So I talked to God as I sat in my lawn swing, rocked in the hammock, went for long walks or listened to the rain during my escape. I wrote pages full of prayers. I won't bore you with letting you in on all of my very personal journal entries, but I'll share this one.

Journal Entry

Someone told me they were going to pray harder. What does that mean? I firmly believe that when people pray, God hears the desires of our hearts, and I believe He definitely intervenes on our behalf. But I'm realizing that after you've done all you can do—in my case, it's been surgeries, physio, chemo etc.—it's still up to God, and my future is in

> *His hands. So what does it mean when people say "keep fighting", or "fight for all you're worth" or the Christian way of saying it, "be strong and courageous"? After you've done what you can, there's a real need to stop "fighting" and relax and be weak enough to be quiet and crawl into Jesus' lap and be willing to say "Your will be done." It's realizing He loves you even more than your husband, your children, your sisters, your mom, or anyone else here on earth. And He knows the desires of my heart—to be here for a long time yet. But He has also given me a new fresh perspective on life—and on death. I have a hunger for heaven I've never had before. And a hunger for a closer, deeper relationship with Him. I guess what I'm trying to say is, instead of letting the terror that I know lurks deep down inside come up and take over, I'm realizing that crawling into Jesus' lap isn't weakness, or mean I've stopped fighting. I'm learning it's absolutely a very intentional choice. It's the difference between living in the fear and letting it pervade your life so you can't really enjoy anything anymore, and living with peace, enjoying every moment, looking for God's hidden blessings—those precious moments or situations that you just know have been God working out the details.*

A quote I found in one of the "cancer books" I took with me to read on my escape: "When you have laboriously accomplished your daily task, go to sleep in peace. God is awake." (Victor Hugo)

Chapter Six
More Chemo

Chemo Round Three

Email update to my team

Subject: Pre–chemo Round 3

Thanks for praying... Yes, I had some trouble with my port again today, but it worked after some blood thinner was injected into it. The blood work came back and it's a go for Friday. The dr. said my blood count was very, very good. I don't know why but I needed to cry and feel sorry for myself on the way home, though. I think just being in the oncology dept. and talking about it all day has a depressive effect and I needed to get that out of my system. But I had my little pity party and gave it back to God again and it's all okay. After my treatment on Friday, I'll be halfway done my chemo—YAHOO!

Thanks again for praying.

Love,
Sherri

EMAIL UPDATE TO MY TEAM

Subject: Chemo Round 3—Chemo crash

This session of chemo was not fun today and the joy of the Lord has disappeared. Both Ron and I woke up with heavy hearts today and shed tears before we even left the house this morning. Why now? I don't know. I think this has all just taken its toll and today was one of those fall–apart days. I was trying to pull it together all the way to the hospital and thought I was doing okay, but when we got to the treatment room and the nurse came in, I had trouble speaking because of the tears. These nurses are not fazed by it and I was given some tissue, and meds asap. I felt much better once the happy pill took effect and we got started on the chemo regimen. It all went well and we are home. I've had a nap and I feel better but still teary and joyless. I am officially halfway through my chemo treatments now and that should make it a celebration of a milestone, but I'm so tired of this that it clouds my thoughts. I know that I still have 3 more to go and then 5 weeks of radiation after that. It's already been 6 months since this "unrequested journey" started, and in the beginning, the dr. told me that in 6 months I would be finished with surgery and treatments and be on the "other side." But that wasn't a realistic picture and I'm very much not done yet. I'm telling you this to help you get a picture of how we're doing today, and we very much need your prayers and support.

Thanks,

Sherri (and Ron)

EMAIL UPDATE TO MY TEAM

Hi Everyone,

I thought I should 'fess up—I've kind of been in hiding, because I was feeling like I had let people down. It's kind of crazy how stupid my mind works sometimes. I'm a people pleaser—there, I've admitted it...that's the first step toward healing. I'm just kidding. This isn't a new insight at all. ;)

What happened with my last treatment is that it was really a very low day for both Ron and me, and when I wrote about it on Friday and asked for prayer, you responded and God answered above and beyond. I can only say that I was doing amazingly well after having had a chemo treatment and I honestly thought my body must have adjusted to it. My kids were home for the weekend and we had a great time because I was doing so well. I even went to church on Sunday morning—which, by the way, was so good for my soul. I literally felt like I was wrapped in a big bear hug by the church family. The words of encouragement from the church people were like a boost of adrenalin to get over the hump of the halfway point of the marathon and see the finish line more clearly.

On Sunday night, I knew I was crashing. The headache started, I was getting achy, my taste distortions ramped up, and I had nausea. It was so discouraging and I felt like I needed to retreat into hiding. I've been fighting the side effects since then but I've been getting progressively better. Just a bit of a headache this morning, and I'm thinking about eating some breakfast. So I think I can safely say that chemo 3 is behind me now. My week of low blood–count and germ avoidance starts today.

Thank you to the people who have been caring for me and my family in such tangible ways. That warm banana bread last night was amazing (from what I could taste) —thanks, neighbour.

I have a few extra prayer requests that are weighing heavily on my mind and I thought if you have time, could you add them to your list?

- Lindsay is experiencing more of her arthritis/fibro symptoms as she begins her last trimester of pregnancy and could use some encouragement and prayer.
- Jessie is also needing prayer. She has had complications throughout her pregnancy and has been warned that the baby will be early. We are rejoicing that so far the baby is healthy and we're praying that it can stay inside to grow a bit more and that these complications won't be serious.
- My girlfriend is slated for her first chemo treatment today. I remember how held I felt when I went and I want that kind of peace for her as she begins her chemo phase of recovery today.

Thanks.

Love,

Sherri

Chemo Round 4

Email to my team

Subject: Pre–Chemo Round 4

Hi everyone,

I can't believe it's that time again. I've really enjoyed this past week–and–a–half with relatively no side effects except for the fatigue. I've had a chance to see many of you and that was so good for my well–being. I don't feel ready to go for my next chemo treatment but then I don't know if anybody is ever ready for a chemo treatment. ;)

Tomorrow at 9:15 I have an appt. for the blood test, which will determine whether or not my blood count is high enough to go ahead with the treatment as scheduled. I would appreciate extra prayer for this because so far my port has not cooperated as it should and it takes a few tries before it works. Last time it took 2 injections of blood thinner. So it would be great if it could work right away, but if not, that I would be able to relax and not get too anxious about it. After this, we wait for 2 hours to see the oncologist to find out if it's a go for the treatment and discuss the next treatment.

I've negotiated to postpone my treatment until after the long weekend so it is slated for Tuesday, Sept. 2nd at 9:30. I'm requesting prayer for this treatment because I will be starting a new chemo drug, which I will be receiving for the next 3 treatments. It's common for people to have an allergic reaction with this drug and I have no idea which side effects I might be dealing with. It sounds pretty scary. But I did reasonably well with the first chemo cocktail and so I'm hoping and praying that this will go smoothly.

Please pray also for Ron and my family. This journey is getting old and I can tell we are all tired of this and running out of gas.

I'm telling myself that after Tuesday, I will only have 2 treatments left. And I can't even begin to worry about the radiation treatments after that…

Thanks again for your encouragement and for lifting me/us up in your prayers. Thank you also for continuing to hang in there with us.

Love,

Sherri

Email update to my team

My appt. went very well today. Thank you so much for praying. I felt reasonably calm—you can ask Ron!—and MY PORT WORKED!!! I actually said Hallelujah. The bloodwork took 15 min. this time instead of the 45 min. it took the last time. My blood count is down a bit which apparently is to be expected but it is still in the normal range and so we are not postponing treatment. We went over all of the possible new side effects of the new chemo drug with the oncology nurse and even though it sounds bad, I know that after Tuesday, I only have 2 more treatments left and I feel right now like I can do this.

So we're heading off to the lake tomorrow after Ron finishes his service calls, and planning to stay until Monday. Treatment 4 is at 9:30 Tuesday morning.

Thanks again for praying. The nurse wanted to know what was different today—why did the port work? I said I had asked for extra prayer specifically for it to work. She smiled knowingly. Isn't God awesome? He cares about the little details.

Thank you Lord.

Love,

Sherri

The drug I was switched to for treatments four, five and six is called Taxotere (Docetaxel). This treatment started with an IV round of Benedryl—to prevent an allergic reaction—and then the Taxotere. To minimize possible side effects, which may include nerve damage to extremities, I was given frozen mittens to wear on my hands to decrease the blood flow and lower the chance of the drug being carried to my fingers. Interesting stuff. I had no allergic reaction, so the treatment was drama-free and shorter than the previous ones.

Email update to my team

Subject: Chemo Round 4

Hi everyone—just a note to say thanks again for praying for me yesterday. This was my calmest treatment so far. It is amazing to think that I only have 2 more to go from here. I couldn't have done this without your prayers and encouragement and support through it all. You'll never know how appreciative I am of this. You have taken me to my Father's throne even when I wasn't up to doing it in my own strength.

The port worked well again and we were home by 2ish. After a 2–hour nap, I was feeling pretty good, so we decided to go out for dinner to celebrate our 30th wedding anniversary. Yes, I had a chemo treatment on our anniversary! I wore my wig outside of the house for the first time. I am getting tired of the curious stares of strangers and I'm afraid someone is going to get hurt one of these days. (That bad Sherri still wants to come out sometimes!) We had a great evening. I had a solid night of sleep and woke up this morning feeling as if I was well enough to go to a job—if I had one! I'm waiting anxiously for the other shoe to drop—it can't be this good. A bit of a headache and feeling off kilter a bit, but nothing major. I know based on the past treatments, my worst days are days 3 to 6, so I know it could come yet and I'm planning for it. I'll let you know. But for now, I feel like this is bonus time and I plan to enjoy it. I have some painting to do for my grandbabies. ;)

Thanks again for praying me through. To God be the glory…

Love,

Sherri

Email update to my team

Subject: A real update

Hi everyone—I could use some extra prayer as I'm battling new side effects from the switch in the chemo drug. I was doing great right after the treatment on Tuesday and that was a bonus. Now it's a battle. I'm dealing with extreme muscle and joint pain all over my body but mostly my lower back and down my legs. I also have a headache and mouth sores. Not fun, and really difficult to sleep. Please pray that this will subside soon and that I can be brave and cope with it.

Thanks,

Love,

Sherri

Email update to my team

Subject: Real responses

Thank you so much for the real responses tonight. I was thinking that most of you would be out and gone on a Friday night, but I have been surprised by the responses we have received. You are being faithful and we appreciate it so much. There are times when my own prayers seem like so little and feeble and same old that it doesn't seem to matter anymore, but I know that when you pray for us, you are knocking on heaven's door and He hears our collective prayers. Your encouragement tonight has been overwhelming and a new reason to cry—but tears of renewed hope and renewed strength to get through today and tonight and not worry so much about the future.

So thank you very much.

Sherri (and Ron)

Email update to my team

Subject: Turned the corner

Hey everyone—thanks so much for your prayers. When I woke up yesterday morning, after an uninterrupted 4 hours of sleep, I felt like I had turned the corner. It feels like it's been a long week but when I look at it realistically, I've only been "sick" for about 4 days. I'm not great, but much better than I was. My mouth sores/taste–distortions/after–taste yuck are worse than they have been after any prior treatments, but the muscle aching and joint pain is much better now. The headache is also much better. So thanks again for praying. I was able to go to Jessie's baby shower yesterday and genuinely enjoy myself.

Sept. is as bitter–sweet month, isn't it? It's saying goodbye to summer and getting back to a more regular schedule for a lot of people. With my life like this, my schedule is different than it's ever been before. No deadlines, no job to go to, no kids to chase after…I should be enjoying this life of leisure. But my heart craves normalcy. I want all that normal stuff. And then I wonder why… because it validates who I am and justifies me being here?? I know this questioning comes now in Sept. because "normally" I would have gone back to school after the summer break—14 years of working in the school system does a number on you that's hard to shake. So on top of the physical battle of beating this cancer and getting through chemo and all that it entails, I'm fighting an inner battle—in my mind and heart. I'm not depressed—just questioning my existence—which I think is also part and parcel of the wakeup call to reality that cancer imposes on you. I say imposes because this wasn't something I asked for or wanted. But even an imposition can end up being an unexpected blessing and I really think that when all is said and done, I'm not going to be the same person I was. Look out, world!

Sorry for the rambling…too much time on my hands!

Love,

Sherri

Chemo Round 5

Email update to my team

Subject: Pre–Chemo 5, Yay!

I didn't think I would be excited about a chemo treatment, but 5 seems like the one right before the very last one, so in a warped way I'm excited to get it over with so I'll only have one more after it.

So today is "blood test and meet with the oncologist" day. My appt. is for 12 noon for the blood test, and it worked so well last time, I'm asking for prayer again that my port will cooperate and it will go smoothly. If not, that I will be calm about it. Also, pray that my blood count will have recovered sufficiently so that my treatment won't be postponed. I had a trip to the emergency on Tuesday evening to treat a UT infection, but it's much better now with antibiotics. Please pray that this won't be a complication that could postpone treatment, too.

If I get the green light for treatment, I'll start on the steroids tomorrow and have the treatment on Wed. at 9:30 a.m. Please pray that the side effects might be less this time. The fevers, headaches, and body aches were rough to handle and lasted way too long. I've had a pretty good week now and have almost forgotten the aches of the two weeks before.

It's my birthday today and we are going out for supper with my children to celebrate tonight after my appointments. It's funny how your perspective on life and birthdays changes when you're on this cancer journey. I'm absolutely thrilled to be able to celebrate getting older!

As a special birthday gift, and with His special sense of humour, God has decided to bless me with a very small but significant sprinkling of new baby peach fuzz on my head this week—and it's mostly dark hair—not white! How crazy is that!! I don't know if it's here to stay, but it's kind of cool to know that He sees and knows and cares about every little detail of what we are going through as His children.

Hope you have a great day,and thanks again for praying for me and my family.

Love,

Sherri

Email update to my team

Subject: Pre–chemo 5—Didn't happen yet

Well, yesterday didn't go as I would have hoped, except that I stayed calm, which is what I asked you to pray for. ;) My port didn't cooperate and it took a while and a few attempts and finally a blood thinner injection to get things moving. A blood sample was taken and then we saw the doctor an hour later for the results. My blood counts weren't great but good enough to go ahead with the treatment tomorrow morning.

Now I have another problem—my neck started bothering me last night and this morning the port area and up to where the catheter is in my neck is swollen and painful. I've called the oncology dept. and I'm supposed to go in for them to check it out as soon as possible. I'm not running a fever, so that's a good thing.

Please pray that this won't be a serious setback. Pray for peace to prevail and for wisdom for the people taking care of me.

Thanks for all of the birthday wishes you sent my way. I wasn't expecting that—it wasn't why I mentioned it. But very nice... We had a wonderful birthday dinner with my family (minus Cait). The only non–wonderful thing about it was that the fire alarm went off twice while we were there and by the time we got back inside the restaurant, the food was cold. But now I get to enjoy it at home.)

If all goes well today, treatment 5 should take place at 9:30 tomorrow morning.

Sherri

Journal Entry

October 1, 2008, 1:04 a.m.

I can't sleep. I have the terror ache in my stomach. I've had a wicked last week–and–a–half. Since my birthday last Monday, it's felt like I'm on that tunnel of doom roller coaster. My health is out of control and I want to get off this ride.

It started with the usual pre–chemo appointments. But my port was acting stubborn again and the blood test didn't go well. After several attempts of flushing, blood thinner was injected through the line and then it behaved. But it didn't feel right. By Tuesday, my neck was sore and swollen and we went back into oncology to get it checked out. The first thought was a blood clot and the second was infection. The nurse also gave me the information that my chemo would be cancelled anyway, due to my blood–count being too low from the blood test the day before. The decision was made to redo the blood test to check my counts as well as infection, and I had an emergency visit to the ultrasound dept. to determine whether there was a blood clot in the line or in my neck. Well, no blood clot was found and the test for my white blood cell count came back with my numbers being high enough to go ahead with chemo the next day. Another blood test was done just to be sure about the infection—one from the port and another from the arm to compare them to see if there was infection brewing in the line. I was sent home knowing that treatment would go as planned the next day.

The next morning—The swelling had gone down quite a bit overnight so everybody thought that was that. We proceeded with the treatment but I complained about the burning lasting longer than usual and it was chalked up to the fact that the port had been used so often in the past few days.

Email update to my team

Subject: Chemo 5 is done!

Yes, everything went very well today. I had no fever this morning and my swelling had improved a lot so chemo went ahead as planned. No big reactions yet. Last time it took 2 days for the side effects to hit so my plan right now is to go to bed and sleep these past few days off so I'm ready to take on the side effects.

Thank you so much for all of your prayers and your heartfelt concern. I can feel it in my soul.

It's hard to fathom that I only have one chemo treatment left.

It's been a humdinger of a journey. Thanks for sticking with me and my family so far.

Love,

Sherri

Email update to my team

Subject line: "Down for the count"

Okay, I'm pretty low tonight. I know I'm in chemo and it's not supposed to be fun but this last round has kicked the legs out from under me. I think that the complications of my neck and port being swollen before chemo has compounded the problem and I'm not feeling good at all. I'd like to ask for prayer for the swelling to go down so I can be more comfortable. And I need patience to deal with not feeling well. I could use some extra prayer tonight. I thought about not emailing because I feel like I'm needy and pathetic but then I realized that's exactly why I need to ask for prayer. Ron and I have prayed together and on our own but God's telling me it's time to rally the troops.

Thanks,

Love,

Sherri

I was feeling fine when we left the hospital after the chemo treatment but the next morning, my neck seemed swollen again and when I checked my port site, I saw that it was quite red. I didn't have a fever so I wasn't too worried. I should have been but I didn't know it. By Friday, I had intense pressure in my head from my port site up to my ear. My neck was very swollen and my port site was angry red with deep purple veins webbing around it up to my neck. I was worried, but I thought if it was an allergic reaction, it would have happened sooner. I waited till 4:00 to call the oncology department to ask about it and the only one left was the nurse who had administered the chemo. She said she was sorry but there was no one left in the department. Everyone had gone home already. She advised me to head to the Emergency department if I was concerned. I decided to tough it out. It could only get better from here. Well, no, not exactly…it could get worse.

My Lowest Point

This weekend was intense. When I look back now, I see it as the lowest time of my entire journey.

I had a visit from an angel this weekend. I don't think she knows this, but her willingness to come over and calm our hearts and minds was such a huge blessing to us. A special couple from our church lives a few miles down the road from us. Ron refers to him as his "Gilfriend." (His name is Gil) They are as close as brothers. His wife, Diana, is a registered nurse and administered some of my Heparin injections (to prevent blood clots) when I needed them after my surgeries this past year. On Sunday evening, Ron called her to ask if she could come over and see if she could figure out some way to relieve my pain and anxiety. At this point I was pacing back and forth, circling around my dining room table like a wild animal. If you've never had serious constipation, you might not want to keep reading. I was in agony and, to complicate things even more, the pressure from the swelling in my head and neck was preventing me from being able to push without feeling like I would faint or my head was about to explode. I had taken all of the prescribed medication and the result was extreme stomach cramps added to my already long list of ailments. I was miserable and actually contemplating suicide. I didn't think I could hang on much longer. It sounds so overly dramatic now but I know that in my heart, that Sunday night, I was just finished with the whole fight and wanted it to be over. This woman sat at our table and calmly listened to our concerns, gave us some suggestions, and then asked if she could pray with us. Her prayer was so honest and heartfelt and touched me right where I needed it. When she was done, I felt like my burdens had been lifted and handed over to the Lord and I would be okay. Thank you again, angel, for being available and willing to be used as an instrument of blessing to us, and to the glory of God.

Things resolved themselves before I crawled into bed that night. I realized later that I shouldn't have been so stubborn and should have allowed others to take me in to Emergency to get some help. Looking back, I know I had an incredible fear of not being taken seriously and it takes so much energy to try to explain what is bothering you. A visit to the ER is usually long and complicated, especially when you need to drive in from out of town. My thinking was that it was just easier to stay home and deal with it.

We headed back to the hospital on Monday to consult the Oncologist, again. I thank God for our Canadian medical system. Can you imagine what all these doctor's visits would cost? We'd be bankrupt already!

Email update to my team

Subject: more prayer?

Hello,

We had another day at the hospital today. The doctors decided it's time to take out the port and they don't fool around, so the appt. to do this is tomorrow afternoon at 2. I've been dealing with the pain and swelling for a week now and so I'm looking at this with relief. Please pray for there to be no complications—I've just had a chemo treatment last week, so the chance of infection is increased and we don't want or need that. I'm feeling better today than I was yesterday so it doesn't seem as overwhelming. I'm still dealing with all the chemo side effects on top of the port situation. Pray that these will subside. Also, that I'll be able to have a good sleep tonight to be ready for tomorrow's challenges. I'm hoping to be a happier camper soon. ;)

Thanks for your faithfulness in supporting us.

We are so grateful for it.

Love,

Sherri (and Ron)

Email update from Ron to my team

Subject: Sherri's status

Thank you!!

We came back from the "procedure" (that's what they call things to give you the illusion of it being something insignificant...I think) and felt a real peace as God was faithful in answering prayers. It went well and we feel like this was a bit of a milestone. Not that we are done, but that the port is out. Sherri already noticed before she left the operating room that she could swallow more easily again and she was able to eat more than has been possible for many days—praise the Lord. I drugged Sherri up (in a good way) and put her to bed...I thought I would take a break from the laundry to send an update and thank everyone for their faithful prayers.

Ron

Another Journal Entry

I'm feeling kind of down and I can't get to sleep. So many thoughts going around in my head. I don't like it when these scary thoughts come, but I know I can't just ignore them and stuff them away. I need to write them down:

- *The babies are coming soon and I desperately want to be healthier and stronger to help my girls out, but now this whole swollen neck complication has messed up my plan.*
- *At this point…and don't tell Ron…I'm almost tired of fighting. I've had so many months of getting knocked down and then working at it to get back on my feet just enough so I can get knocked down again. I'm tired of feeling crappy.*
- *I'm scared. I read on the Internet—yeah, bad me. When the port has allowed a chemo drug to leak out, it can take a long time for the body to repair itself, or it may be irreparable. I don't want my neck to hurt like this anymore.*
- *I'm really, really scared of the next treatment. With the port out now, it will have to be done by IV, which is a big concern but…I'm most scared about dealing with side effects of this awful drug again. What if they are even worse than what I'm dealing with now? I know it won't kill me, but I don't know how much lower I can get. I'm so tired and buzzed from the pressure of the swelling in my neck, and sore and having nerve pain in my legs, not to mention the horrific constipation I survived on the weekend. Oh, yeah, and the fungus mouth that was diagnosed the last time I saw the doctor and…I got my period on the weekend! Wasn't that supposed to stop? How can I possibly manage another treatment—even though I know it's my last? I don't want to let anyone down, and I know my husband and family are cheering me on and wouldn't understand me not wanting to do the last treatment. I know in my head that I'll go through with it. I'm just really, really scared.*

My Prayer

God, I come to you with all of my weakness and fear. I don't feel very much like a victorious child of the King. Please see me and hear me and know that I need you. I'm feeling desperate. I know you love me and care about what's happening to me, but I can't feel it tonight. I'm so tired and hurting. Please take away my fear and replace it with your hope and peace. Only you can do that. You are my Redeemer. I can only walk this valley knowing You are beside me. Hold me. Give me sweet, sweet sleep, and I pray if it's Your will that I'll be better in the morning. I love you and I trust you with my tomorrows—even if I can't feel it tonight.

Amen.

Okay, I think I can go back to bed now.

Email update to my team

Subject: Friday update

Hi everyone—I decided that it was time for an update from me personally, so you would know what is going on. I had the port removed on Tuesday as you already know. Thank you so much for praying me through that. I was so calm—even when I found out in the OR that I would not be getting twilight sedation for this as I had been told. The local freezing was enough, though, which made recuperating that much easier. God gave me another one of those guardian angels who stayed on my left side through the procedure and carried on a conversation with me while the surgeon did his thing. Pain from the incision site has been minimal. The surgeon informed me that the port had in fact been leaking for the previous chemo treatment, which accounts for the pain and swelling in my neck as well as the burns and angry veins in my chest. So since Tuesday, I've been recovering from the port removal, managing chemo side effects, and dealing with my neck. It's been what seems like a slow climb out of the hole. I feel like I'm improving in very small steps, but at least its upward now instead of getting worse.

If I can be honest, could you please pray for my emotional well-being as well as physical healing? Every time there are complications, I feel like God has forgotten how much I want to get better and not have setbacks. I really just wanted to get another chemo treatment out of the way so I could recover from it and then have my final one. My eyes were on the chemo finish line and I didn't see the pothole coming up. So I'm frustrated and disappointed. Again, I know God loves me and is walking through this with me but I don't always feel it, especially when I think I'm being faithful and trying to handle this like a trooper.

Again, thank you so much for your prayers. I have relied on your faithfulness in holding us up to the Father.

Sherri

Chapter Seven
Needing a Cure

Run for the Cure Weekend

It was a hard, tough weekend. In the past few months, my family had been planning to participate in the *CIBC Run for the Cure*—a fundraiser for fighting breast cancer. My daughter Lindsay had been spearheading the project, and the number of "Team Sherri" members was so encouraging for all of us.

The night before the event, I was still stubbornly refusing to think I wouldn't be participating. My sister, Laurie, came to spend the night. She gave me a pedicure and painted my toenails and fingernails a brilliant shade of pink—matching her own—in anticipation of the Run the next morning. It felt great to be pampered but even better to know she was there not only to join the other team members in raising money for such an important crusade, but as a means of personally encouraging her older sister in her cancer fight. On the morning of the run, I realized I was just too sick to go. It was so discouraging, but a decision I needed to make. My very pregnant daughters and their husbands, my son and his girlfriend, and about twenty–five other people would be there expecting us to do this with them.

This is the email I asked Lindsay to read to the group:

Team Sherri,

I am so disappointed that I'm not able to participate with you this morning. I started running a fever overnight and just don't think I should be out in public today. My heart and thoughts are with you as you collectively not only hold me up with your support this morning but also helped to raise money to combat the very reason I can't be there. Cancer sucks, and it just makes sense to work together to rid this world of it. I've been so overwhelmed by the response to Lindsay's idea to do this run. You've raised quite a bit of money, but you've also shown me and Ron and the rest of my family that you are behind us and supporting us, which is so appreciated. Have a great run or walk and enjoy brunch together.

With much love,
Sherri and Ron

Email update to my team

Subject: You are my Sunshine

Hi everyone,

I'm sorry to send so many updates in the past week. Are you prayered out yet? "Oh, no, not ANOTHER email from Sherri!" Hey, no one promised this would be an easy road that you have chosen to walk with me, right?

I wish I could report that everything is rosy and good. It's been a long weekend with trying to will myself into feeling and acting healthy. The truth is that I'm not, and I think I'll need to go back to the hospital today. I'm running a fever off and on, and my neck and ear area are still inflamed and causing me much pain. A major disappointment for me this weekend was having to miss the Run for the Cure event on Sunday. That was a tough decision but I know it was the right one. I felt a bit better later in the morning and we ended up going to meet most of the Team Sherri supporters for brunch. They all cheered me up so much and gave me so much hope to keep fighting. Thanks to those of you who were there.

What can I say? Please keep praying that this complication will get sorted out and that I'll be feeling better very soon. I need for the doctors to figure out what is going on for my own peace of mind.

I hope you can find or spread some little bit of sunshine today in spite of the rainy weather outside.

Love,

Sherri

Something is Wrong

We went back to see the doctor on Monday and he gave me an anti–inflammatory drug to take down the swelling and relieve the pain in my neck, head and ears. I went back in on Wednesday and the swelling was down and the pain was better, but I still felt a lot of pressure in my neck and head, and felt like something wasn't right. I could feel and see that my arm was getting purplish if I tried using it. The nurse and the doctor tried to convince me that I was better and the blood flow was normal and everything was okay. But I cried and said, "Help me—this isn't okay." I had debated doing what I did next, but decided that if it came to it, I would. So I showed the doctor pictures of my pregnant daughters and told him I had so much to live for and wasn't ready to give up. I needed for him to grasp that I was not just another cancer patient and he needed to take my concerns seriously. I think he got the picture. He said in order for us to know if we could go ahead with the last chemo treatment, he would need to schedule another ultrasound.

Well, the ultrasound was done the next afternoon, but I had a funny feeling about the technician's body language. She didn't talk much and went over one spot a few times. When she explained that she needed to do the other side of my neck for comparison, I had that sinking feeling. It was pretty much confirmed when she told me I should go back to oncology to wait for the results. Why would we need to wait for results if nothing showed up? So we went down to oncology and were told there would be no news for at least an hour. We found some lunch and then we went baby shopping to take our minds off of what could be.

When we got back to the hospital, we knew something was up. We were told that the oncology nurse was just waiting to hear back from the doctor. She came to usher us into an office and told us the ultrasound showed a blood clot in my jugular vein—the catheter from the port had been threaded into this vein in my neck. Now what? I was told that people don't get hospitalized for this anymore, but I would need to have daily injections of a blood thinner for about three months. It was almost an instant relief just knowing that there really was something wrong and they finally found out some real answers. But with that came anger—questions were raging in my mind: "How did you not believe me?" "How long have I had this and you thought I was okay?" I was mad that I had to cry and beg for help but I was glad I did.

I had my first injection in the oncology treatment area. The nurse who administered the injection had tears in her eyes and said she was so sorry that I had to go through this on top of everything else, and she was sorry to have to give me this injection because she knew it would hurt me and leave a bruise on my stomach. I kind of laughed and reassured her that this was not a big deal. I had injections of this drug for the previous two surgeries and knew what I was getting into. As the evening wore on yesterday, I felt myself getting angrier. How much more would I need to endure before this nightmare was over? Isn't it enough to have to go through the surgeries and deal with recovery and the state of my body after them…and then the horrible port experience, having to go through my jugular vein instead of the usual chest insertion…and then chemo treatments? I have successfully survived five chemo treatments. None of them were fun and battling the side effects is not for wussies, but I did them, got through them, and all I wanted was to have that last one and close the chapter on the chemo phase of treatment. Why does life throw these curves at me? What did I ever do to deserve this? I just want to be a healthy, happy wife and mother, and now a grandmother. Is that too much to ask for?

These are some of the verses from the Bible that came to me. I was clinging to them as I tried to make sense of all of this…

> I pray that out of his glorious riches he may strengthen you with power through his Spirit in your inner being, so that Christ may dwell in your hearts through faith. And I pray that you, being rooted and established in love, may have power, together with all the saints, to grasp how wide and long and high and deep is the love of Christ, and to know this love that surpasses knowledge—that you may be filled to the measure of all the fullness of God. Now to him who is able to do immeasurably more than all we ask or imagine, according to his power that is at work within us, to him be glory in the church and in Christ Jesus throughout all generations, forever and ever! Amen. (Ephesians 3:16–21) (NIV)

Email update to my team

Subject: Good News/Bad News

Well, the good news is that thanks to an ultrasound I had this afternoon, I now have a much better idea of what is going on with the swelling and pain in my neck area. The bad news is that it is a blood clot in my jugular vein. The treatment for this is daily injections of blood thinners to dissolve it (for about 3 months). I had my first shot this afternoon and I already have one of my angel nurse friends offering to give me the injections at home for tomorrow and the coming weekend, and we'll figure it out after that. I can honestly say that I feel relieved and a bit vindicated because I have been in and out of the hospital often enough in the past 2 weeks saying that there is something very wrong here. It gives us peace of mind just knowing what it is and that it can be fixed. My next chemo treatment would have been this next week, but that has been postponed. I'll see the doctor next week Tuesday to decide if, or when, the next treatment will take place. Thank you so much for keeping us in your prayers. I have felt the strength of you people praying. I know this feels like another bump in the road—a scary bump—but I have peace. My blood–count is up now, and I hope our almost–daily visits to the doctor are over for the time being, so if you're healthy and have time on your hands, I would love to see you.

Love,

Sherri and Ron

Chapter Eight
Happy Thanksgiving

Email update to my team

Subject: Happy Thanksgiving

Hi Everyone,

I didn't feel very thankful when this weekend came. I was so blessed to be able to attend the church service on Sunday morning (after missing church for a few months) and hear what I didn't want to hear about being thankful. I feel quite differently about things after hearing what the pastor had to say, and I'm much more thankful than I was—and happier, too, in the process. I'm not glad about the complications I'm dealing with, but I've had my eyes opened to the wonderful things God has placed in my life that I am so extremely thankful for. After stating the obvious—my husband, my children, my children-in-law, my soon-to-be grandbabies (and I am in no way understating how important they are to me, how much I love them and am so very thankful for them) and my extended family, I have to say that the support and encouragement I've received from this support team and my church family has blown me out of the water. When I started this little team of cheerleaders (aka prayer and support people), I had no idea how much you would come on board with me and my family and play such a huge role in keeping us in your prayers and in encouraging us—some of you on a daily basis and in very tangible ways. I just wanted to take this opportunity to say thanks in a big way. So…

Thank you.

And now for the rest of the story…

We saw the doctor again today, as we hadn't been able to see the doctor on Thursday when my blood clot was diagnosed. We asked many questions and confronted him as to why the blood clot hadn't been found sooner, etc., and we felt he was quite open to our questioning and responded with an apology. We won't be dealing with him again because we are being referred back to the head oncologist/hematologist next week, but we feel like we were heard and maybe patients coming after me will be taken more seriously. I played the ultimate card by showing him pictures of my family and my pregnant daughters, and told him this is what I have to live for and I need to be able to trust the medical staff to take care of me and ensure I am there for my family. I'm also thankful for the nurses (friends) God has placed in my life, who volunteered to take out their frustrations by coming over to jab me with needles this weekend. The St. Anne Home Care nurse started coming in today to give me my daily injections of blood thinner, and it gives me some reassurance that a medical person will be in daily contact, as this is a dangerous location for a blood clot. I have more peace now that we've asked our questions until our appt. next week with the oncologist. The pressure has let up quite a bit, so I'm not as light–headed as I was, and the pain and swelling have lessened considerably. Please continue to pray that this clot will not dislodge and will continue to heal. I would also like to ask for prayer for the medical team, as decisions will need to be made next week re: chemo 6.

Hope you all had a bit of turkey this weekend and were able to enjoy some time with family and friends—except for y'all Americans! You'll be partying next month.

May God bless you, and thanks again for being there for us.

Love,

Sherri

Email update to my team

Subject: Doctor's appt. tomorrow

Hi everyone,

I have a blood test tomorrow morning at 8:30, and then an appt. to meet with the head oncologist/hematologist at 10:00. Please pray that we will have some clear answers for our questions. It is still uncertain whether or not I will be having my 6th chemo treatment. It is tentatively scheduled for Thursday, but with the blood clot complication, we are hanging in limbo. Pray that we will be confident and clear in our questions and that we will feel satisfied with the answers. It feels like so much is riding on trust, and our trust level with the doctors is kind of low right now. Please pray that God will supply us with the knowledge and peace we need to make informed decisions tomorrow.

Thank you for praying about the daily blood thinner injections. They seem to be doing their job, and I feel much better than I did. The injections themselves are becoming routine and the colours on my belly are spectacular. The Home Care nurses coming in to do the shots are amazing and so diligent about checking my medical condition. It makes me feel well taken care of.

I'll let you know what comes out of tomorrow's meeting.

If you read this tonight, please pray for us to be able to sleep tonight. The possibility of the 6th treatment and worrying about it is weighing on both of us.

It's so great to know people have my back.

Love,

Sherri

Let's Recap

It's been a few weeks since I've documented anything in my life. I feel kind of guilty, because so much has happened and I might have forgotten some of it already. Sometimes writing in the thick of it is better because you can feel the passion and emotion of the moment.

I guess the biggest recent event in my cancer journey saga

is that I was referred back to the head oncologist, and he decided it was too risky to attempt another chemo treatment. So chemo treatment 6 was cancelled. This brought a bittersweet resolution to the chemo phase of my treatment plan. I was tremendously relieved, because I have no idea how I would have survived another treatment with the blood–clot complication to deal with, as well as chemo side effects, never mind the ordeal of trying to do the treatment using an IV when I know how hard it is to start an IV on my one good arm. I was very relieved, and yet…questions lurked in the back of my head; "Was five enough? Am I wimping out? Will the cancer recur and then I'll be sorry? Did the first five get it all?" The doctor assured me that chemotherapy was adjunct therapy and that the actual cancer had been removed during my surgeries. He said the tests showed there was no malignancy in my body and we could be confident that five treatments of chemotherapy were sufficient. We were told we would move ahead to the next phase of treatment now—Radiation Therapy.

Email update to my team

Subject: Re: my appt. today

I don't even know where to start. It's still sinking in…I'm done chemo. The doctors had discussed my case and reviewed my file and history. When the oncologist came in to see us, he shared the plan with us. He said we could be confident that this was the right decision. So I'm done!

Also, he is switching me to blood–thinner pills instead of the injections, which will take a bit of time and a bunch of blood tests, but in the next week or so I should be switched over. I really had the expectation of doing chemo 6 on Thursday and just didn't know how I could handle it with the blood clot business and injections. This change in plans is HUGE and my mind is still trying to process it. One small thing that it means for me is that the hair growth that I have will continue and I don't have to think about it falling out again! Yay! My energy level can keep getting better and better and I'm not going to be sick and recovering from chemo when my grandbabies are born. If I had permission to jump up and down and dance around the room, I would be doing that right now, but the doctor has given me a list of dos and don'ts regarding my blood clot so I better sit tight for now, but know that I'm dancing in my heart.

So now I'll be waiting for Radiology to contact me about starting radiation and going in for blood tests to get my blood levels to where they should be on pills now instead of injections.

What a huge answer to prayer—and a finish to a milestone. I managed 5/6 chemo treatments and I survived!

Thanks for walking this path with me and carrying me at the times when I was too discouraged to walk on my own. I'm not done yet, but I feel like the biggest battle is over...yeah, it's over...

Can't quite grasp it yet.

Love,

Sherri

A Healthy Confrontation

Before we moved on to radiation, there were a few things I needed to take care of. Moving to radiation meant a radical change—new building, new doctors, new nurses. So I needed to tie up some loose ends at the oncology department at the first hospital.

The one thing that was foremost in my mind was to discuss the past few weeks with the doctor who had been treating me. I felt that he needed to know my thoughts and, yes, I wanted to vent, but my other, more unselfish motive, was to make sure his future patients would be well cared for. We may have cancer, but we are humans who need to be treated with the best care possible. I was able to articulate my concerns and did it well, if I do say so myself. After I had explained myself to him, he ended up apologizing and admitting that a patient would know her own body best, and that he should have ordered that second ultrasound earlier so the blood clot could have been treated sooner. That was good enough for me. What was done can't be undone—the port is out and the leaking chemo drugs had done their damage. I needed to put it to rest and I felt I could now that I had discussed it with this doctor. We shook hands and I forgave him.

The highlight of the appointment for me was the nurse's reaction to what I had said to the doctor. She introduced herself before the appointment and just sat at the back of the room listening to the discussion between the doctor and myself. After the appointment, she left the room and then came back after I had gotten dressed. Ron had gone to get the car from the parking lot, so it was just the two of us. She clapped her hands and told me that what she had just witnessed was the best patient advocacy she had ever encountered. She said I had done such an awesome job of explaining my concerns and without too much emotion—just the right amount to get my point across. She asked if I had experience in advocacy, and I thought about it and realized that my role in the union in my previous job had been advocating for the employees. I guess I did have some legitimate experience. I think the assertiveness training class I took this past year in my HR education didn't hurt either! I felt it had been a very good appointment, which was affirmed when this nurse gave me a big hug as we exited the examining room.

My Chemo Closure

You'll think I'm silly, but I was disappointed that I would have no grand finale chemo appointment. I had a special hat and scarf I had been saving to wear for this special occasion. My daughters, and possibly my sisters, had planned to be there. I wasn't going to wear it anywhere else! It is a bit too festive for me but a great gift from a friend to cheer me up and support me—a golden, glittery set with sequins for that bling effect. I wondered what I needed to do to bring closure to this chapter. We decided to bring flowers to the oncology department the next time we were at the hospital. I was going to the lab at the same hospital for scheduled blood tests, so we knew we would be back. I wanted something happy and bright to cheer up this department because it was situated in the basement of the hospital and had no outside windows. I called it the dungeon. Ron found some warm, sunshiny–coloured Gerbera daisies—yellow, red and orange—and they were perfect. Even the card had a sun on the front. In the card, I thanked this team for being so encouraging and supportive. I had way more complications than I had ever expected during the course of my treatments, and they never treated me as an inconvenience. I could walk in there and be treated as someone special who needed their help. Those warm blankets they spread over me were like big hugs that let me know someone was taking care of me.

This oncology department has since moved to a brand new wing on the main floor of the hospital. It has big windows and everything is new and glorious. Quite the difference from the dungeon area. I was almost sorry my treatments were over, because I wanted to be able to be treated in the new building. How crazy is that! I said "almost!" The nurses hugged me and had tears in their eyes when we presented the flowers and card to them. It really gave me the closure I needed to move on.

Blood–Clot Recovery

I was so very, very relieved I wouldn't be dealing with recovering from chemo treatments while my daughters were in their last weeks of pregnancy or dealing with newborns. I had time to recover from the blood–clots.

The daily injections of blood–thinners were not fun at all, because the dosage was maximum strength to ensure the clots didn't get any bigger or dislodge. This was scary, but I have to say these home care nurses made it so much more bearable. My stomach was colourful, with brilliant hues of blue, yellow and purple at every needle site. The original plan was for me to have these injections for three months, and I had no clue how that would ever work when my stomach was so sore and bruised already. The nurses were so adept at their jobs and kept a close eye on my blood pressure, temperature, etc., just to make sure I was doing okay.

The blood clot problems slowly began dissipating. The pressure in my head comes and goes and my arm still turns purplish depending on how I'm using it and for how long. The port site isn't angry, swollen and red anymore. There is damaged tissue around where it was situated, but even that seems to be healing slowly.

I had a few weeks to recover before I would need to start the next phase of the journey.

Email update to my team

Subject: The next step

Hi Everyone,

Did you think you were done?

Sorry, but I'm not. The next step is about to begin, and I still feel the need for prayer and support through this. I have an appt. this afternoon at 2:30 to have my markings done for radiation. I don't feel ready…when I hung up the phone I was overcome with a rush of emotion. I wanted some time to feel more "normal" before I needed to start radiation treatments. I was told it would be about 10 working days after marking till treatments will start. I thought I should warn those of you who have volunteered to be on my list of potential drivers. Hopefully my grandbabies will make their appearances before I'm locked into treatments every day.

Let me know if you want out of this email group. I know it's been a long journey already and I wouldn't blame you if you wanted out already. When I look back to see where I've come from, I don't know how I could have managed without knowing I had such a group of faithful people standing behind me. God hears your prayers and answers them. I can literally feel the power of your prayers sometimes.

Yesterday I read a devotional that talks about how the Holy Spirit isn't the gentle, huggy spirit we think of when the Bible says He is our "Comforter." The translation of Comforter is actually more of an empowering push that we need to shove us into battle. That made me think that as we trust in Him, He's the one who gives us the strength that we need to go through the battle—whatever battle we are faced with. I know we all have them—some of us are more vocal about it than others. ;)

Love,

Sherri

Chapter Nine

Same Story, Next Chapter

Enough About Cancer; Let's Talk About Babies!

The past weeks have been totally consumed by end–of–pregnancy stuff. My girls both ended up being overdue. I know this has all been God–orchestrated from the beginning, so this overdue business was also part of the master plan. But my poor girls! The upside is we had some quality time together before the babies came. With both of them on maternity leave waiting for babies and me on "cancer leave" waiting for radiation treatments to begin, we had no jobs to worry about! Who knew?!

Baby Number One

My youngest daughter, Jessica, delivered her baby on November 5, 2008. Everyone (but me) thought she was having a boy. I was still holding on to the notion that it would be a girl. I bought two outfits just in case. But it was a girl! Little Chloe Marie (named after her grandma—me!—Sherrill Marie) was born after forty hours of labour. She was six pounds, fourteen ounces, and twenty-one-and-a-half inches long. A string-bean like her mama. It was a tense and long wait for this baby. All of my windows were scrubbed clean while we waited for news from the hospital. We were so relieved when her husband Kevin finally called to let us know the baby had been born. We rushed to the hospital to welcome (and inspect) our new granddaughter and congratulate the new parents. I'm so proud of the way they dealt with, and have adjusted to, this new responsibility and treasure in their lives. Jessica was here for her first trip out of the house with the new baby a week after she was born. I had so much fun introducing my precious first granddaughter Chloe to Grandma and Grandpa's house.

Email update to my team

Subject: Same story, next chapter

Hi Everyone,

Since I wrote my last update, we have become grandparents to little baby Chloe (Kevin and Jessie's) and it's about the most awesomest thing that could happen in our lives, next to knowing that another baby girl is on her way (Geoff and Lindsay's), which will make us grandparents for the second time in very short order. We feel very, very, blessed. Thank you for all the prayers that have gone up on behalf of my daughters. Chloe and her mommy and daddy are doing very well. Lindsay and Geoff would appreciate prayer as they anticipate the arrival of their baby at any time. She is 9 days overdue and her arthritis/fibro symptoms are flared up, so unless natural circumstances prevail, she will be induced soon.

The new chapter, as far as my cancer journey goes, is the one on radiation treatments. I got the call this morning to start treatments tomorrow afternoon at 3:15. I guess they assume we are sitting at home waiting and have no other life besides this cancer world? The good news is that if I get started now there's a very good chance I'll be done by Christmas time, which would be a great reason to celebrate. I'm feeling quite calm about this, although if I could have any control, I would love to wait until baby 2 is born and life has adjusted to some sense of normal. But as I've learned, life is not in my control. I'm not thrilled about knowing that these treatments will happen every day for the next 5–6 weeks and I don't know what they will do to my body. But I do know that I've survived so much already with God's help and the prayers and encouragement of faithful friends and family. I have to trust God to help me get through this new chapter. I have so much to live for! My energy level is much better than it was, and most of the chemo side effects are almost gone—a bit of a lingering headache at times. My blood–clot symptoms are also much better and slowly clearing up. I'm on oral blood–thinners now and the bruises from the injections in my stomach are mostly gone. I have blood tests every week to check my levels and so far the levels have been very good.

Another update I have is that I will be meeting with an oncology gynecologist on Friday to discuss another possible surgery that might be happening. In treating the type of breast cancer I have been diagnosed with, the usual course of action is to take a hormone–suppressing drug for 5 years after treatment is finished. Because the number one side effect of this drug is blood clots, and because of my presenting problem and history with blood clots, the oncologist is thinking that it would make sense to surgically remove my ovaries and possibly the uterus also instead of controlling my estrogen production with this drug. This would shift me into instant menopause. It would also make it possible for me to take a different drug that wouldn't have the risk of blood–clotting. I'll have more information after meeting with this doctor on Friday.

Thank you for sticking with me and letting me know that you don't want out of this commitment to pray for me and Ron and our family. Your prayers and encouragement are so invaluable. I hope none of you will ever be in this kind of situation, but if you are, remember to be vulnerable enough to ask for this kind of support. I can't imagine doing this alone. No one should ever have to.

My main prayer requests would be for peace, again, and to trust God at an even deeper level. I know that the plans He has for me are good ones, but I have trouble trusting and having faith that His good plans are better than the ones I want. My deepest desire right now would be for there to be no unexpected side effects during radiation or any new complications. I hope and pray that is God's plan, too.

Love,
Sherri

Chapter Ten

Radiation Therapy

Not Yet...I Need More Time

I know I'd been waiting for it and yet dreading it at the same time. I went to the Manitoba CancerCare building two weeks ago to get "markings" for my radiation treatments and was waiting for the phone call to let me know when my treatments would start. They had prepared me that it would take ten working days to get set up. Well, yesterday was nine days, so I knew it was coming. I just wasn't prepared to start the very next day!

The good thing about getting started now is that I think there's a very good chance I'll be done by Christmas! It's funny how your own expectations and deadlines change as your circumstances change, and your mental calculations fluctuate and flex as needed. I remember thinking at the beginning of summer that chemo would take a certain amount of weeks, and checking the calendar and making plans accordingly. When the appointments aren't in your control, and complications come, the calendar changes and if you're too set in your mind that this is the way it is going to be, you better be ready for the depression and discouragement that comes with your inflexibility. I've had some down times about this and totally understand it. So when this phone call came and I realized they wanted to start tomorrow, which is now today, I had to mentally rearrange my internal calendar. In my mind, both babies would be born and settled in. My daughters would both be adjusted to their new mommy roles and doing fine before I would get locked into my daily radiation treatments. I was so concerned that my appointments would interfere with me being available to help them with their newborns.

Lindsay, my oldest daughter, in addition to her rheumatoid arthritis, has also been fighting fibromyalgia with chronic fatigue for the past few years. She managed amazingly well with her unexpected pregnancy, but was in pain now from carrying this extra weight on her body. I wanted to be there for her to help her out. I was holding on to my expectations of what a mother should do, or what I wanted to be able to do for my daughters. I sure didn't expect to be dealing with cancer treatments during this very special time in their lives. Under the heading: "Things I Can't Control."

So, that day, I headed in one direction—to my first radiation treatment—while my oldest daughter had an obstetrician appointment where she and her husband made important decisions about inducing this baby. Odds were that she could have been in labour while I was being radiated. Happy thoughts.

Email update to my team

Subject: About today

Today went okay. When we went into the actual radiation treatment room, the technician was telling us what was going on and it seemed different than what I had been told, so I asked a few questions. He decided to get a hold of the radiation oncologist to talk to us. So we went back to sit in the waiting room. A little while later someone came to tell us that the doctor wasn't available, but the head of the radiology department would come to answer our questions. Nothing like going straight to the top! We had to wait longer but it was worth it. He had actually taken the time to review my file and had it with him, including some of my CT films. He showed us the pictures and explained everything so well. He had so much knowledge and it was reassuring to be able to ask questions and have him answer them. I'm much more confident, now, that these people know what they're doing and are doing what they think is best to make sure I'll never need to do this ever again. The chances of recurrence are so vastly lower after radiation that it would be crazy for me not to do this and do it the way they seem to think it needs to be done. The scary thing is that it raises my chance of more lymphedema in my left arm because they are radiating some lymph nodes in my neck area, but it makes sense to do it after talking this over with the doctor today. I think I'd rather deal with lymphedema than have another cancer recurrence. The first treatment was done after our discussion and it was like an x-ray. The only difference is the humming sound when the radiation beam is on. They are beaming on 3 locations and the beams last about 20 seconds each so the actual treatment is only 60 seconds in total. What takes a lot of time is the positioning of my body in relation to the radiation laser machine because the technicians are very accurate about it and came to check measurements 3 times during the treatment. That's a good thing. No sense radiating something that shouldn't be radiated! I got my schedule for the next week and all of the appointments are later in the afternoon, so it should work for Ron to drive me.

Lindsay had her appt. this afternoon and everything is fine—baby's heartbeat and mommy's blood pressure. The doctor says her body is so ready to have this baby. She was surprised to see her at the appt. because she thought for sure that she would have delivered by now. So anytime now—how many times can you say that?! She will be induced very soon if she doesn't go into labour in the next day or so. Yay! Another little baby girl. How blessed can I be? I feel so very, very lucky.

Love,

Sherri

Random Radiation Ramblings Journal Entry

I've been having some random thoughts, now that I've started radiation, and I thought I would get them down on paper before I lose them. I had a tough time with relaxing during my first treatment. As I was lying on the "table" (a narrow, hard surface with a sheet covering it to camouflage the truth), I heard the heavy door at the other end of the room slide and bang shut. Everybody else left the room so they wouldn't be radiated, and left me all by myself in this big, cold room. I had this machine pointed at me hovering just above me, but right in my sight line. I wasn't allowed to move. The last words spoken to me were, "Now hold very still." So it was me and this machine staring at me. As I was lying there, I decided to make friends with the machine. If we had a standing appointment to meet together every day for the next five weeks, we should at least be friends. I know it probably sounds pretty silly to you, but it was the one way I knew to cope with this situation and it helped me to relax. I stared at the glass of this machine and could make out a friendly, happy face and realized in my heart again that this was all meant for my own good—not to harm me but to give me a future. (Jeremiah 29:11) When I came back the next day for my second treatment, I felt like I knew this machine already and, as it was positioned up above me again, I looked at it and almost felt relieved to see a familiar face.

The other line of thinking I've needed to process is a surreal feeling that this isn't happening to me. I've realized I'm using the denial strategy to cope with the treatments of cancer and putting up a wall to block out my feelings and pushing through what I need to get through. Maybe this isn't a bad thing. I don't know. I'm not a psychologist. Maybe it's time to talk to someone who understands—or a professional? As I was sitting in the waiting room be-

fore my first radiation treatment, I felt out–of–body—as if it wasn't actually happening to me. As I walked with the technologist to the room where the treatments would be taking place, I didn't feel connected to myself. As if I had gone to my happy place. I don't know if that makes sense at all. I've had thoughts before about how stuff like this happens to other people, and now that I'm in the thick of it, I wonder how it got to this. How did this happen to me? And then the reality hits—yes, what is happening to me is too much to handle, so I am trying to block it out. It's much easier to think of someone else dealing with cancer and praying for them in a third–person way, and not having to think about the reality of what is actually happening. Unless you've been through it personally, you just don't know—and I don't blame anybody for that, because why would you want to know before then? It's just too scary and puts you in touch with your own mortality, which can be a terrifying thing.

So last night, I crashed. I felt like I'd been holding back the wall for a while already. Probably since my blood clot complications. I was just in survival mode then and felt like I was on autopilot. I remember crying a bit with the relief of knowing I was finished chemo, but it was like I had stopped letting myself feel at that point. Yesterday, I felt again. A dam broke and I had a really necessary healing cry. My words while I was crying were of desperation. "This has gone on too long! I just want my life back!" I don't really want to process what I was saying because I think it was too raw and real. Don't make anything more of it than a woman who just had enough and craves normal living—just wanting to be healthy and not having medical appointments and pills and treatments dominating her life, and wondering and worrying about her future. It felt good to be real. My poor husband Ron had a very wet shoulder. He's been so good to me and didn't judge me for falling apart.

Chapter Eleven

Another Baby!

Baby Number Two

I had two radiation therapy treatments and then baby number two, Briony Evangeline, was born eleven days after her cousin. Another too long delivery—if I had had hair, it would have turned gray or been pulled out from the anxiety and worry! Baby B arrived after twenty–five hours of labour on November 16, 2008. She was eight pounds and also twenty–one–and–a–half inches long. Briony's heart rate dropped significantly during pushing, and she wasn't breathing when she was born. An NICU (Neonatal Intensive Care Unit) team resuscitated her and she was in observation for a while before the new parents could hold her. Lindsay and Geoff were obviously shaken up and distraught by the ordeal. We were all so relieved when we found out she was absolutely fine.

Briony was named after her father's English heritage,

and Evangeline was a tribute to my mother, Eva. She was a gorgeous newborn with blond hair and chubby cheeks. These little girls made their entrances to the world tough on their mommies (and daddies!). My grandma–heart is so full of love and pride and admiration for my daughters, who fought so valiantly through their long pregnancies, labour and scary deliveries.

I had no idea of the depth of love and connection I would have for my new little grandbabies. From the minute I held them, I had an immediate feeling of family—a sentimental, deep, intense bond. These little girls will be part of our family forever and ever. It's an awesomely good feeling.

Email update to my team

Subject: Roller coaster ride

I haven't been able to figure out a better analogy for my life this past year other than that of a roller coaster ride. Huge ups and downs. Most of you know that our 2 beautiful baby granddaughters have arrived in the past 2 weeks. Both girls gave us ulcers while we waited and prayed for their arrivals. They are very different and are both very beautiful babies. No bias from this grandma! Meeting and holding these perfect babies has been the huge "up" of this past month.

I guess in a way, starting radiation was also an "up" because it means that treatment is happening. I was at peace when I went for my first treatment but I think it was more of a mind thing—going to my happy place and not letting myself feel. By the time I got home after my second treatment, I could feel that a crash "down" was imminent. I cried in Ron's arms and I think my exact words were, "I just want my life back." But the crazy thing is that I don't want that old life that rushes off to work every day and worries more about if my clothes are coordinated with my shoes than about the person sitting next to me in a waiting room or seeing the pictures in the clouds. You know what I mean. There are things that are so much clearer and more important to me now. I'm living in HD instead of the old analog!

So now my life is centred around going to appointments for radiation every day for another 5 or 6 weeks and fitting in trying to be of some help to my girls with their new babies. So far I have no side effects other than a sore arm and sore neck, but this is because of holding them at awkward angles for so long during positioning for the treatments. The technicians seem to be having some difficulty in positioning me and it takes up to 30 minutes for them to be happy with the accuracy of the positioning, but the actual radiation treatment takes 20 seconds each for 3 angles so that's 60 seconds total for the actual treatment. I'm glad they are being so cautious and accurate, but my affected arm and my neck (behind the ear where the blood clots are in the jugular) aren't quite as happy about this. I was told not to expect any side effects for at least 2 weeks after the start of treatments. The main side effects are soreness of the skin where it is being radiated and a lowered energy level. Nothing to report so far—I was tired before I started ;) and some people don't actually get any side effects. That would be absolutely awesome and you can surely pray for that, but in reality, I'd just like to keep them to a minimum and get through this without complications. According to my calendar, my last treatment will be on Dec. 23rd, but I've been told that this can be thwarted because of machine breakdowns or unforeseen delays. Could you please pray that this schedule could carry on as planned?

So, ready for another "up?"

I saw the gynecologist yesterday for the results of my last pelvic ultrasound and to discuss possible surgery in the future for treatment after radiation. This doctor told me that the cysts in my ovaries and uterus are very small and very benign—no other cancer in my body!! The oncologist at the Victoria Hospital had told me this after my CT scan, but when the ultrasound results came back, he was a bit sketchy and wanted this gyn. to take a look at the results. So that was a huge relief. Again, I didn't realize how this was weighing on me until I got the results and felt that weight lifted. Thank you, God. I will possibly be having one more surgery at the end of January to remove my ovaries so that I can take the recommended drug for the 5 years of post–treatment. This is still up in the air. We need to ask more questions about this so we can make a more informed decision. You can pray for wisdom in making this decision and also being able to trust the experts. I really don't want another surgery if it isn't absolutely necessary.

That's where I'm at right now. I'm actually feeling quite good physically and emotionally right now. But I've only had 3 treatments and I know this is going to get old very quickly—not only for myself but also for Ron. He wants to be able to drive me for treatments as much as possible, so he is working 1/2 days and then coming home and picking me up and driving me all the way back to the HSC for my treatment. So far they haven't been the "drive around the block twice and she's done" treatments either, so it means parking and sitting in the waiting room for me. So my prayer request for radiation treatments is for perseverance and stamina to get through this and that we will stay healthy so we can maintain the schedule and "git 'er done."

Please keep my girls on your prayer list too. Lindsay is struggling with recovering from a tough delivery as well as arthritis symptoms. She was started on some arthritis meds in the hospital. Jessie is doing well but is quite isolated where she is and I can't get out to help her as much as I would like to now, with my treatments dictating my life.

Thanks for praying. Sorry this turned out to be such a long update. I didn't realize when I started that I had so much to tell you!

How's everybody else doing? I have time to pray as I lie there and "hold very still."

Love,

Sherri

My Radiation Break

On the weekend Lindsay was in labour and delivering her baby, I didn't know I would have some time off from my radiation treatments. When I went back on Monday for my next treatment, I brought in my brag book and showed off my new, beautiful granddaughters. I still think this is a great way for the people who are caring for you to realize, if they haven't already, that you have a life and that you matter to other people—ultimately, that you are a person, not a number.

The technicians had trouble with my positioning again, as they had with the initial appointments, and the treatment took way too long. I could sense some frustration on their parts. I couldn't understand why my treatments were taking so long.

People would come and go out of the room with that big steel door sliding open and then clanging closed behind them. They would adjust me a little bit this way and a little more that way, and talk amongst each other.

I finally asked if they could please talk to me so that I would know what was going on. I told them it was scary for me to lie there not knowing what they were saying or doing. This seemed to be a new experience for them—to have someone ask for clarification or want to know what they were doing. Do all radiation patients just lie there and not ask questions?

I was asked to come in earlier the next day but again, they didn't say why. I realized later that they wanted to be able to have the CT team and doctor on hand to check this and fix it if possible. Maybe they didn't want me to worry about it or they just didn't think that it was my problem to deal with. I don't know. But if they had just explained it to me! I'm a big girl, and it made sense once I figured it out for myself.

We came in early and yes, it was a problem again. I was sent back to the CT simulation room where some other techies worked on my positioning for a long time and obviously with my radiation computer program. I had an intern in that room who I didn't appreciate. I'm sorry, because I recognize the need for them to learn, but not at my expense. I had been through enough! He tugged on the sheet underneath me to reposition me, but his tug was too hard and violent so it shook my neck and head. I was still recovering from the blood clots in my neck and I had been so careful about not moving it quickly, as I had been advised. I thought to myself that this would be crazy dying here on this table from an embolism an intern dislodged because he was too eager. The older technologist realized what he had done and reprimanded him. It was better after that.

Finally, they said I could get up off the table and get dressed. By that time I was really hurting from having my arm up above my head and my head turned for so long. I was happy to be able to move again.

Email update to my team

Subject: The roller coaster is broken

Yeah, I had a downer of a day at my radiation appointment today. I didn't get my treatment today. The radiologist recommended having me go back to the CT simulation and checked to make sure my tattoo marks were aligned correctly. I ended up being on the CT table in position holding still for another 45 minutes while different doctors and techs came in to do adjustments and measurements. Someone said today that I was brave for baring my soul in this morning's email. Let me tell you, that wasn't all I was baring for most of the afternoon!

Finally, I was informed that this just wasn't working and I was going to have to have a mold made for my future radiation treatments. This means that I have to go back tomorrow morning at 8:00 to have a plaster cast made of my chest and neck area. This will be used to make a hard plastic mold for me, which should be rushed and ready by Thursday. I have to go back on Thursday for another round of CT simulation and markings. Then it will take a couple of days to redo the computer programming for my treatments. Hopefully, I can start again on Tuesday or Wednesday of next week if all goes as planned. They said that using this mold will position me correctly, more accurately and more quickly for the rest of my radiation treatments.

Forget what I said this morning about doing alright physically and emotionally. My arm and neck are very sore now and I imagine tomorrow won't be easy either with the plastering. But I'm mad and sad about having complications again. This means that radiation will NOT be done by Christmas as I had hoped.

I realize that in the scope of everything else that I've already survived, and the rest of my life, this complication is not a big deal, but it feels like it is right now. Thinking back about my prayer request from this morning, I guess it hasn't really changed. I need prayer for perseverance and stamina to finish this course. I also need to regain that inner peace to keep fighting.

Thanks,

Sherri (and Ron)

I was informed that I would need to have a mold made and a completely new computer program drawn up to continue radiation treatments. The early eight o'clock appointment the next morning was to make a cast of my upper body. Ron was able to be in the casting room with me, and I have to say the guy doing the casting was great. He was funny, although his jokes were lame. He said he had casted one man who was a priest and in a hurry to get to a meeting. He was wondering how he would explain to the others at the meeting why he was late. The cast guy told him he could always say he was out getting "plastered." Before he started, he told me he had twenty–eight years of experience doing this and it would be done quickly and efficiently. I believed him and this was one of the better appointments in my cancer journey. It could have been awkward, as I was lying there exposed again and feeling very vulnerable, but he was absolutely professional about it and made me feel safe.

The next step was to have the cast made into a plastic shell. Usually this takes a few days, but we were called in for a fitting the very next day. It was perfect and markings were put on it and I went for another CT scan so the computer program could be set up. As I lay there on the table for the CT scan, I began to realize I had exposed my bare breasts to a lot of people in the past week—let alone in the past year! I told the radiation tech that he was the twelfth person I had exposed myself to in the past three days. He laughed and said I should expect to be doing this to at least twelve more people before this was over. Not what I wanted to hear!

After this was done, I was told they needed time to redo the computer program, and normally this takes about two weeks, but they would rush it and try to get me started again in the next week. I didn't realize what a blessing this would be. It was actually a gift because for the next week, I didn't need to plan my days around my next appointment and instead, I could concentrate on my daughter coming home from the hospital with her new baby. She needed help after a rushed delivery, breastfeeding issues and her arthritis flaring up. I was so glad I had recovered sufficiently from the blood clots and still had some energy, and the side effects of radiation were not evident yet so I could feel like I was able to be of some assistance to her.

Our son–in–law's mother, who happens to have been a labour and delivery nurse/midwife in her past career, was coming out to help with the new baby for a week. The timing ended up to be just about perfect. I helped whenever I could, and when the call came to resume radiation treatments, she had arrived and was able to come to the rescue. Lindsay developed double mastitis and was in rough shape with this infection. She needed help, especially when Geoff went back to work the second week after baby Briony was born. I'm not sure if she was as happy as we were that their house is pretty much en route to the hospital where I was having my daily radiation treatments. We stopped in for a baby fix quite often and it was nice to have tea with the other Grandma in Briony's life.

Email update to my team

Subject: FYI

Hi—just wanted to let you know that I had an appt. this afternoon for a final marks verification for my radiation mold and it went very well. I had my fourth treatment right after that and it only took about 10 minutes. Yay!! Thank you for your prayers and encouragement during this frustrating time. I had a good talk with God yesterday morning and basically asked Him to show me that He was still with me and cared about my delay in treatment. I know it sounds silly to ask God to do that because He should really be focusing on bigger issues! But He totally answered my prayer. About 15 minutes after I prayed, the phone rang and it was the HSC letting me know that I had an appt. today to get started again. Isn't that crazy! I knew the minute this person asked for "Sherrill Hildebrandt" that it was the radiation dept. and I was filled with relief in knowing I could get started on my radiation therapy, but mostly for God showing me again that He is in control and I can trust Him.

So let's pray for no more road blocks or pot holes in the treatment journey—and if they do come, that I'll have the strength and grace to adjust my expectations accordingly.

Thanks again for your prayers,

Love,

Sherri (and Ron)

Having the new mold was amazing. Instead of trying to adjust me on the table for forty–five minutes for every treatment, it was usually more like ten minutes for the entire treatment.

Here's the email where I described to my mom and sisters about what the treatments were like with the mold:

You Asked About Radiation?

The mold is solid–hard, clear plastic and it fits over top of me and gets bolted down onto a hard, plastic board once I'm positioned on it lying on the table. It holds my arm up over my head and covers the left side of my head, holding my head with my face pointed to the right. It covers all the way down my chest and my sides and reaches down to about my waist. I asked about what they did with it after my treatments were done, and they said I could take it home if I wanted to, so I'll show you sometime (or if you take me for my appt. sometime, you could come in and see it). It is supposed to be "comfortable" but honestly if you can picture how I'm positioned, it's not really, but it's doable and I try to go in with a good attitude. I do get kind of claustrophobic and feel like I'm hyperventilating when I've been bolted down for any length of time. I can't move at all except for my fingers and my legs. That's when it's time to go to my happy place—right now it's thinking about the babies! There is a small foam piece for my head and they put 2 facecloths under the right side of my face to take the pressure off where my blood clot place is behind my ear. I also have a big triangle foam wedge tucked under my knees to help with my lower back.

Radiation doesn't hurt at all and if I didn't recognize the hum of the machine when it's working, I wouldn't know when it is happening. When they are happy with my positioning on the table, everyone leaves and a huge, heavy steel door closes behind them with a loud scraping sound. I feel very alone even though there is usually music playing. Today it was some country music so that didn't do much for me. So far my arm and boob are sore and getting a bit stiff, but I don't know if it's from the treatments or from holding babies. :) It would be early to have any side effects, but who knows? The skin is still holding up and I haven't noticed any difference—no burning yet.

I don't think that there is any way I'll be done by Christmas with the delay this past week. I'm just glad they got me back in so soon. So far I've had 5 treatments. That's a week's worth of treatments, if anybody is keeping track.

The technicians there are really nice and seem to care a lot about me. That's worth a lot. I told them today that they could call me Sherri now that we know each other so intimately! The reason it's still taking a while is they are still taking pictures to verify positioning every day. They told me that tomorrow they just need to take one more picture and then the treatments will just be the actual radiation, which only takes about 5 minutes.

Thanks for asking for details about radiation. It's actually therapeutic for me to tell you about it.

This weekend has been tough for some unknown reason. Maybe it's a culmination of relief of the stress of having the babies born and having radiation treatments figured out. I don't know. Ron has a headache, which he gets when the stress level is down. He's so great when the adrenalin is pumping, and he can keep going for a while, but when the drama is over, he crashes by having a bad headache. This happened after every chemo treatment. He would be awesome for the treatment and for the days after when he was still in high alert to help me through the side effects. But when I was feeling better I could anticipate the crash. I can't blame him and I don't fault him for it. Better men would have gone running in the opposite direction long ago.

Chapter Twelve

Ode to Joy

We stayed home from church this morning. With Ron's headache, I thought we had a good excuse, but I know now it was God's direction. We had a time of sharing over coffee and we shed some tears that had been locked up for a while. I was feeling quite down when we went to bed last night. I'll admit it—I spent too much time on cancer websites yesterday. The statistics are still not good enough for me to breathe easy and face the future confidently. The fear and panic start to rise and I can feel it in the pit of my stomach. It's not a good feeling. I think that having the grandbabies was a tremendous distraction from the cancer journey, but yesterday I came face to face with the reality that I am battling cancer. I'm not just going to radiation because it's what the doctors have advised me to do and it's not just another treatment that I have to slug through and get over with. This is actually a battle for my life and my future. I can live in denial and plod through what

I need to do to get through to the other side, to a point, and then every once in a while the stark truth rears its ugly head and the fear creeps in. "Am I doing enough? Am I doing the right things? Do the doctors know what they're doing?" I kind of lose perspective in that I really don't have much control over this at all. I can do everything right and trust the doctors but in the end, either there is no more cancer or I could die in a car accident tomorrow. Now there's a happy thought.

So instead of attending church this morning, we watched a TV message given by a pastor we used to watch months ago when I was recovering from surgeries. His message was titled "Ode to Joy."

His points were:

1. We have the freedom to choose our attitude and how we will respond to the situations life throws at us.
2. Joy comes from within, not from the pursuit of happiness.

This was just what I needed to hear. What I gleaned from his message was that I can choose to enjoy every day no matter what the circumstances might be that I am dealing with. The funny thing is I told Ron when I woke up this morning that I needed to start changing my attitude and enjoying every day I have left in my life—whether that time is short or is many more years. I have to learn to live with the fear of the future because I don't think I can honestly say there's any way I can stomp that down. I think it's more realistic to learn to live with the uncertainty—knowing I'm doing everything medically possible to fight the cancer and my prognosis is good. Not great, but good. I can also be encouraged that medical research has brought cancer treatments so far in the last few years and even though people still die from it, many more are living quality lives because of the advances. This gives me hope and joy to face the future without the burden of worrying.

Some random things I want to remember about this radiation chapter:

- The little girl who came with her mom and grandma who was having treatments and played in the waiting room. She spilled water on herself and the floor every time, and then worked hard to wipe it up with napkins. She was a story of faith. Her mom shared how Faith had been born prematurely and had been in grave danger. A C–section was performed, which saved her life. By the way, I met Faith's grandma in the hallway on my last treatment day and she told me she was done. I shook her hand and congratulated her. She seemed like an old friend even though we had never talked to each other before.
- The mom and daughter in the waiting room. The daughter was the one having radiation. You know who is there for the nuking when they are wearing the "happy blue gown." This mom was a wreck. She came in swearing at her daughter in some other unfamiliar language, but in some universal way, we know when someone is angry and cursing no matter what the language is. She kept going and going. I don't know what she was so mad about. I would think the daughter had much more right to be complaining. Although, the woeful parking accommodations around the medical centre are enough to make anyone mad!
- One of the therapists was a wonderful young woman and would have been one of my "young adults" in the Sunday School class I taught at my church, had it been a different situation. We just seemed to connect and it felt good. She looked

out for me and was genuinely thrilled to see me when she was assigned to my unit. She became engaged over Christmas and couldn't wait to show me her ring and tell me about it. My son Aaron became engaged shortly after this and it sounded like they were planning their weddings for the same weekend in July.

- The young intern. Oh, how I loved to hate him. Just kidding…kind of. He was too young to be an intern, too green, too young to be seeing me in my helpless, vulnerable naked–chest state. I asked for him to be removed from caring for me. Too awkward. Too close to my own son's age. I felt sorry for him. I was concerned the rest of the radiation team would be upset with me but instead they supported me and made me feel like it was okay to request this. I was instantly less anxious about future treatments.
- The automatic door that opens into the CancerCare building from the main hospital atrium. Our routine was to disinfect our hands as we were leaving after treatments and then Ron pushed the automatic door opener button so we wouldn't need to touch the germ–infested handle. One day, he pushed the button and there was a woman on the opposite side of the door and as the door opened she was being squished between the door and the wall. The door doesn't open very fast at all. We didn't know why she didn't think about moving out of the way but she just stood there. She wasn't really trapped at all but she hadn't thought about just removing herself from behind the door. We were trying to keep a straight face

but some chuckles leaked out and she remarked out loud, "and they think that's funny?" Heck, yes. These days, we get our amusement wherever we can find it!

- The awesome treatment nurses who took care of my radiation burns. When the skin started opening up, there seemed to be genuine concern and compassion. When the unit treatment nurse was sick and away, the doctor's assistant took over and made sure I was being checked and had my dressings changed. They also kept us stocked with bandages and anything else we would need to do dressing changes at home.
- My sisters coming to a treatment. They met us in the waiting room and saw where I got changed. We all went for coffee at the hospital cafeteria after, and it just felt really good to have someone other than Ron see where we've been coming almost every day for too long. They were able to experience sitting in the same waiting room where we have spent so much time and mingling with other cancer patients who are also dealing with having their bodies being radiated. It's kind of sobering, and for me it brought a sense of belonging—strange as that may seem. I knew that every person in a happy blue gown sitting in that waiting room was fighting the same killer monster as I was. Kind of a morbid club. I felt totally okay without a head covering—sitting there, bald and in a blue gown, because everyone could either relate or understand.
- Having Geoff and Lindsay's home open to us. I was able to relax and lie down if I needed to. It

was a quiet oasis in the middle of the city and I appreciated it so much. Last night we ordered pizza for supper and I was able to hold baby Briony for a while. I think I was too tired to carry on much of a conversation and we left early, but I was very thankful that they were home and we were so comfortable spending time together. We've stopped in quite often and I've spent time there in–between appointments during radiation treatments and while Ron had work to get done. Much appreciated.

Email update to my team

Subject: I'm positively radiant

Hi everyone—today is a momentous occasion—not just because it snowed so much and the roads are terrible in the city! Today was my 15th radiation treatment, which marks the 1/2 way point for my treatment plan (25 regular treatments and 5 "boosts"). It feels kind of good to know that I'm at that point and kind of disappointing because I thought I would be done by Christmas and that's not going to happen. I was told today by one of the therapists that my skin is holding out well for being 1/2 done. I'm starting to use the 2nd step lotion—a hydrocortisone cream—to help with the itching and burning in some spots. Generally, I'm starting to swell and hurt where the radiation is being directed but so far it is quite bearable.

My prayer requests for this leg of the journey are:

- for a positive attitude—daily visits to the "cancer building" are exhausting physically but also take their toll mentally and emotionally. The instability of my schedule since I started treatments also takes its toll. I thrive on schedules and organization so this has been stretching me in many ways, which isn't necessarily fun. Trying to manage the treatments during Christmas and New Year's will be a challenge.
- for continued health. I realize that I had some control over who I chose to be in contact with during chemo, but now I'm with people in waiting rooms every day and it scares me

because I can't imagine doing radiation and being sick at the same time.

- for strength and endurance to finish the course. I'm so tired of this…need I say more?
- for peace to prevail. I'm starting to look ahead and sometimes the fear takes over. I just don't know what my life will look like. I know now that I will probably for sure have another surgery coming up at the end of Jan. so I know already that I'm not done after radiation is over.
- for my skin reaction and swelling to not get out of hand. I really don't want this to be harder than it needs to be… again…please Lord, no complications. Also, my left arm is starting to hurt more with the same nerve and muscle pain that I've dealt with after surgery. I think the radiation has made it worse again. I could use some prayer about that, too.
- for enough energy to enjoy the holidays and enjoy being with people—especially my little grandbabies. These baby girls have been God's gift to me and my family. They bring so much joy as we snuggle and cuddle with them and burp them and rock them. They are just starting to smile and coo and make funny faces. I love being their grandma.
- for safety on the roads.

I keep thinking of all of you people who are keeping me and my family in your prayers. I pray for you, too. It's a special kind of give–and–take situation. I think it's the way we are supposed to be. In all of this, God sends reminders that He is caring for us and aware of every detail.

In Him,

Sherri (and Ron)

The radiation treatments were not completed by Christmas. They were actually postponed because of Christmas. I had a treatment on the 24th at 1:30 and then had a break from the 25th to the 28th and resumed again on the 29th. I completed the regular treatments on the 30th and then started the boost treatments on the 31st. I had January 1 off, resumed on the 2nd and now it's the weekend and I'll go back next week for three more treatments. My schedule for the next week has a sticker on it—a cartoon character wearing a graduation cap. I told the therapists that's what it feels like and I think someone thought it would be funny to put that sticker on my schedule. I brought my plastic shell home in a garbage bag on Tuesday and one of the therapists said I should consider it a trophy.

Email update to my team

Subject: My Christmas wish

I've been fighting sending this email because I don't want to be "Debbie Downer" at this festive, merry time. But my son told me last night that if I don't ask for prayer, people feel bad because they don't know when they could have been praying. So here goes—I saw the radiation oncologist yesterday because of my burned skin. He called it an extensive burn and now I have heavy duty burn cream and dressings to put on it. Ron was given a crash course in caring for me so that it won't get infected. I have one more regular treatment today and then 4 days off, with 2 more next week and then I'm done these treatments. I start on the 5 boost treatments on the 31st, which will affect only the incision area. And then I'm done and can heal. My prayer request is for no infection. Apparently that seems to be the biggest concern now, along with the pain of the blistered skin. (So much for the "mild sunburn skin reaction" that the radiation information sheets say you might get with treatment!) I'm also getting quite tired from the treatments and driving in to the HSC almost every day. Please pray that I can enjoy time spent with my family and extended family.

Thank you for praying for me.

That's my Christmas wish.

Love,

Sherri

After the twenty-five regular treatments, I needed five more boost treatments to the actual incision site. There was a scary bit of time on the day I went for my first boost treatment. At that point, I had dressings covering the worst of my radiation burns and burn netting holding the bandages in place. During regular treatments, I was allowed to keep all of this on underneath my plastic shell. Now the therapists asked me to remove the bandages so they could mark the area being treated. When I took the bandages off, there was a collective gasp in the room and I quickly realized this was not a good thing. One of the therapists said they would need to call the doctor to come down to check on my burns and let them know how to proceed. I wanted to cry. I had some idea of how bad my burns were and now I was petrified that he would tell me they needed to heal more before we could go ahead with the treatments. When he came in and looked at my skin, his comment was, "Well, that's quite toasted." I held my breath…and then he said it was okay to go ahead with the boost. I was so relieved. It was a bit tricky to figure out how to tape my breast over so the angle was right for getting at the incision site, because my skin was too raw to handle putting tape on it. But between the therapists, myself and Ron, we came up with a solution—using the burn netting. I just held it in place and it worked. What a relief to know we could continue on schedule instead of having another delay.

A Side Story

At about this time, I received an email regarding another cancer patient—a man from the town where we live. He's about my age and he was diagnosed with cancer about two months after I had begun chemotherapy. It rocked the town because that made it three of us—myself, my girlfriend and now Jim—who are all middle–aged and fighting cancer in our little town. The email said Jim was not doing well and the aggressive chemo and radiation he had been enduring had done nothing to stop his brain tumour and it had actually tripled in size. He had a doctor's appointment the same afternoon I started my boost treatments, so there was a real possibility we could run into them at the CancerCare building that day. Oh, my heart hurt for them, and my prayers were going up to intercede for this man's life and for strength for his wife and kids to bear this.

The day after…we met them in the hallway as we walked into the CancerCare building just as I had predicted. What a reality check for me to once again stare this killer disease in the face. He didn't look well. Unsteady on his feet, tired eyes, face swollen from steroids, the classic chemo bald head. They had just come from a meeting with the doctor and there was a possibility of a second surgery. A small glimmer of hope.

Update: Jim didn't make it. He fought hard and was a soldier to the end. We had a real bond knowing we were both fighting the fight. When we met with Jim and his wife, we made inappropriate cancer jokes that anyone else would have been horrified to know we were laughing about. But it was so good for me to be able to do that with a fellow cancer buddy. My heart broke for his family when he went into palliative care. He went to be with his Father in heaven after getting one of his last wishes—a ride on an ATV. The wonderful nurses caring for him made that happen.

After he died, I had a fresh realization that heaven isn't a bad option. It is the ultimate healing.

Email update to my team

Subject: Last treatment!!!

Hi everyone,

I wanted to let you know that it is confirmed that tomorrow will be my last radiation treatment. YAY!!!! I want to say a HUGE thanks for all the prayers that went up for me and my family through this radiation time—especially during the Christmas season. I managed to enjoy getting together with family and friends, which was something I wanted to be able to do, and go for my treatments in the middle of all of it. Even though tomorrow is the last treatment day, I still need to ask for continued prayer for healing and recovery. My burns are "acute" and I'll be needing dressing changes for a while yet. Ron has not only been a great chauffeur and companion during these treatments but he is also gifted in nursing—who knew? There has been no infection so far and healing is coming along. I've reached a new stage of fatigue, so I'm coping with that too. My next big hurdle will be surgery planned for Feb. 4th but I don't want to worry about that yet. We are hoping to celebrate finishing up radiation soon. I need to heal a bit more and get some energy back first but we'll let you know.

Thanking God for having cheerleaders in our lives,

Sherri (and Ron)

Radiation Graduation

Today is my last radiation treatment. I saw the doctor yesterday and he confirmed I will be done today. The burns are healing and the boost treatments haven't really changed the skin where the radiation is being directed. It will be a huge relief to have treatments done. I started in October when I had the markings and tattooing done. It feels like a very long time of driving in to the city for treatments and having my life on hold. By the time I have recovered from my next surgery, it will have been a year. Last night, as we sat looking at each other over supper, I realized that with radiation being done, I can actually start looking for a job. I had an immediate physical reaction to that. Huge butterflies in my stomach and the room swayed a bit. Weird. After dreaming about it for so long, I can finally get on with my life, but I asked Ron, what do I want my life to look like? With cancer treatments done, I can reinvent my life. I don't have a job to go back to and the world is out there for me to re–explore and re–discover. Why am I so scared?

I went to my last radiation treatment and it didn't feel any different from any of the other treatments. Same cold hands and butterflies in my stomach. But as the familiar hum of radiation filled the room, I could feel myself losing control of my emotions. I tried to calm myself and concentrated on the words "keep it together." I even traced the patterns of the familiar leaves on the ceiling with my eyes to distract myself as I listened to the hum. But as I heard the heavy, radiation–proof door slide open after the hum ended, I started sobbing an ugly sob. It was a surge of emotion that came from deep inside and wouldn't be quieted anymore. I felt so silly and yet there was nothing I could do. It was a reaction I wasn't in control of. The therapists helped me sit up and handed me a tissue and then turned away from me. I saw then that two of them were crying, too. It was just a minute or two of unbridled emotion for me and I regained my composure quickly. I thanked the therapists and there were hugs all around. I also was able to show off my oldest grandchild and my daughter as they came with us to help celebrate my last treatment. My other grandbaby and daughter had accompanied us the day before. I saw two of the therapists from the regular treatment unit as we left and I was able to thank them and say goodbye. It was a fitting end to this stage of the journey.

Radiation treatments were over, but dressing changes were not. My husband cared for me, and together we nursed my fried skin back to health. My "mild sunburn reaction" (as the radiation information literature puts it) was in actuality very raw, oozing skin that peeled off in chunky layers to expose delicate, red, new–baby skin underneath. It's absolutely amazing how the human body heals itself. It didn't take more than a week to see a huge difference. Two weeks after the last treatment, the new skin was healthy and, although it was still sensitive, I could wear a bra with some bandages for padding. I saw the radiation oncologist after that and he was very pleased with the healing and said he was encouraged that there were no incidences of infection.

The day after I finished radiation, I read a passage from a book that talked about a guy who was being released from jail. He says, "I want to rejoin life in the real world but I'm scared I won't fit in." I read it again and realized what he said made so much sense for me, too. That's exactly how I was feeling.

Chapter Thirteen
Decisions, Decisions

Another Surgery? Decisions to Make

Email update to my team

Subject: Important decisions to make

Hi everyone,

I am writing to ask for prayer for this morning at 9:30. If you get this email after that, I'm sure God can regard it retroactively. :) We are having a meeting with the medical oncologist we initially saw in June. He is in charge of my case and today we want to discuss future treatment. He had recommended a surgery for me before I even started radiation, but we have our questions and doubts about it now. So we are meeting with him and decisions need to be made as far as surgery and hormone treatment medications.

Please pray for my own, and Ron's, wisdom and clarity of mind for making decisions as well as trust in the doctor and peace for whatever decisions are made. Also pray for the doctor to give us wise advice and take the time to hear our reservations without taking it personally.

I've been quite worried and anxious about this lately and need to "get my act together." Please pray that I can give it up and be at peace and go into the meeting with confidence knowing God is beside me and taking really good care of me.

Thanks,

Sherri

Today was decision day. I had an appointment with the medical oncologist to discuss and decide on the prophylactic bilateral oopherectomy that he had already deemed necessary. This means taking out both of my ovaries and my fallopian tubes, even though they are healthy and happy. After seeing the gynecologist, I had reservations because she questioned whether or not it was necessary. The more research I did on it, the more hesitant I was about it. I sent the oncologist a fax with all of the questions I had been saving up. My reasoning was that it is so hard to get in to see him, so I wanted to make the most of our time together. I was thinking that if he was able to see the questions I had before our appointment, he would be able to answer them with forethought instead of "off the cuff."

At the appointment, he told me he had read over my questions, and using this fax sheet as a guide, I asked my questions and he took the time to go through my entire list. I felt heard and understood for the most part. After further debate and with his expertise and knowledge, the decision was made to go ahead with the surgery.

It was a blunt reality check for me once again. He basically reiterated my chances of survival using statistics to back up what he was saying. He rehashed the gory details of my cancer—stage, grade, size of the tumour, etc., and what the percentages were of recurrence. He told me how my odds were changed by surgery, chemo and now radiation and then explained how much more they would improve if I would have the surgery. He advised that this surgery is necessary because it would stop the production of estrogen in my body and estrogen is what feeds this type of breast cancer. This would give me the same outcome as if I would have taken the anti–hormonal drug Tamoxifen, which is the most common long–term treatment of breast cancer. I can't take this drug because the number one side effect is blood clots and with my history of having two blood clot episodes already, it's not worth the risk. I had a blood test that told us that even though I haven't had my period for four months, the level of estrogen in my body is still too high to say I am post–menopausal. This was also part of the decision–making process. The treatment drug the oncologist would like me to take instead of the Tamoxifen is an aromatase inhibitor called Arimidex, but I must be post–menopausal to take it. If I would take it now without being post–menopausal, he said there would be serious adverse effects such as lesions on my liver. That's actually all I heard. There were more side effects, but that's the one that stuck in my head. So now that I have all of the facts, I will go ahead with the surgery. I don't want to, but I will. Again, I want to live and I have so much to live for, why would I say no to something that will significantly raise my odds for survival?

Now that the decision is made, I should be at peace. But I'm not. The removal of one's ovaries before one's body is ready for them to be non–functioning apparently has repercussions. When you go through menopause naturally, your body has two or three years to get used to the idea and adjust accordingly. When you have this surgery, you are flung headfirst into instant menopause and the symptoms have the possibility of being more intense. I will be looking forward to hot flashes, mood swings, body aches and other lovely things I've only heard other women talk about. I can't take hormone replacement therapy for the obvious reasons—higher risk of breast cancer. Lovely. Can't wait. And yet I have to keep in mind that I am choosing life. By not having this surgery, I'm not choosing at all. I'm letting the cancer choose. And that's not happening, so I'll let you know how it goes…

Releasing my own desires…this is the battle of the mind when you're dealing with cancer. It's so difficult to give up the control you once thought you had in your life. You're giving up so much, too much. Sometimes I sit back and think about my life before cancer and how much it has changed in the past year. And life isn't stagnant so it's changing all around me, too. My family has changed with the babies' arrival, friends have moved on, relationships have changed, my own thoughts about what my future might hold has changed. There are times when I am on my knees begging for some stability and security. As I put it, "Stop this cancer treadmill so I can get off. I'm too tired to stay on it anymore." But the deeper vein that flows through all of it is that as much as I would like to, holding on to my dreams and desires is too hard. The pressure of trying to remember and then be like I was before is too heavy. The hurt of not being able to follow my dreams and ambitions is too painful. And when I decide to let God help me carry my burdens and surrender my life and will over to him, it is freeing and I can "rest in peace."

This is a bit morbid, but it reminds me of something we participated in at a funeral many years ago. The young, disabled daughter of close friends of ours passed away, and after the funeral, at the gravesite, balloons were given to the mourners. After a prayer was said for her spirit to be free with Jesus, we released our balloons as a final goodbye to Allyn. It was also a metaphor for the release of all of the burdens that were associated with her—the pain she endured in her lifetime and the commitment and perseverance her family laboured under in caring for her. They were free to remember the good times and release the tough, not–so–fun memories.

When I pray on my knees to surrender, I release my own balloons.

Chapter Fourteen

One Last Thing...

Surgery Number Three—The Prophelactic Bilateral Sapillingual Oopherectomy

Email update to my team

Subject: Reminder about surgery

Hi again. This is your friendly reminder about my upcoming surgery for tomorrow morning. Thanks to those of you who remembered and expressed your commitment to pray for me. My biggest concerns about this surgery are not actually for me—some members of my family are having a hard time with me going under the knife again. I think the tally of everything that has transpired this past year is just too much and they simply don't want to see me hurting again. Please pray for the joy of the Lord in their hearts. Only He can give us peace of mind and hope for the future and confidence in His love and care. I know that He loves me and is very aware of what I can handle and the amount of strength He can give me. He hasn't failed me yet.

Please pray for there to be no complications and that the surgery will be able to be done laproscopically. Specifically, that the IV insertion will be uneventful and successful without any extra attempts, blood pressure will be stable so I can get pain meds after the surgery, no nausea, no infection afterward, and especially, no blood clots...and anything else you can think of that might go wrong!

I will need prayer for peace in the morning. We need to be there by 7 a.m. and surgery is slated for 9. It is supposed to be day surgery unless there are complications. :)

Please also pray for Ron (and my kids) during the day.

Thank you so much. Hopefully this will be the last surgery I'll need in this journey.

Love,

Sherri

I was to be at Admitting at 7:00 in the morning on the day of the surgery. Several things happened that morning which caused frustration and disappointment for both Ron and me. This was not the hospital where I had my previous surgeries. No one informed us that the day surgery unit at this hospital was a lockdown unit and Ron was not allowed to be with me. We arrived on the fourth floor and saw that there were locked doors and a window barricading the entrance. I was instructed to pick up the phone and talk to the person on the other side of the window. She said that Ron could leave now and that I would be coming in through the door and he would be notified when he could come pick me up. We looked at each other incredulously. After our year of being a team in fighting cancer—through every surgery, chemo treatment and radiation appointment, we were about to be forced to disband our partnership and each go our separate ways. It was an awful, sinking, desperate feeling of panic. How was I supposed to do this by myself? We kissed and said goodbye and he watched as the door opened and I was let in.

I realized again as I walked by myself through the doorway that this was actually quite significant. This cancer journey is my own. As much as I have had the support and felt the love and concern from others and know without a doubt that people are praying for me and God is watching over me, this is my own journey. My husband has been a pillar of strength for me and I don't know how I would ever have managed to do this without him. But in the end, it is still my own journey. So I gave it over to God and asked Him for the peace that only He can give and the strength to endure this by myself. He heard me and I didn't panic. He gave me the peace to wait by myself for another two–and–a–half hours before I was finally taken to the OR.

The time after surgery is a blur to me. Somehow I found myself at home and I knew Ron had been at the hospital to pick me up, but there is a big blank in between. Six hours after he said goodbye to me at the locked door, he was able to see me and take me home but he has no idea what transpired after he left me earlier in the morning. No one talked to him or gave him any information when he came for me. I was pushed in a wheelchair back out of the locked doors by the elevator and he wheeled me out to the vehicle. I remember the doctor coming to see me after the surgery, but I couldn't comprehend what she was saying so she said she would come back after I was more awake. The next thing I knew, I was given my bag of clothes and told to get dressed because my husband was coming to pick me up. My IV was taken out but I hadn't been to the washroom successfully or been given anything to eat or drink. After we arrived home, we found papers in my backpack with discharge instructions regarding my care and a prescription for pain killers. We had no idea when I had last had any pain medication or what I had been given. It was all disturbing. I don't remember most of it but I know Ron was quite upset about it all and after I had time to wake up and process more of it, I also became concerned.

I had a follow–up appointment with this doctor six weeks after this surgery and I had a truckload of questions to ask—starting with wanting to know why no one told us Ron wouldn't be able to be with me for this surgery.

> Email update to my team
>
> Subject: It's all good
>
> Hey everybody—I thought Ron emailed you yesterday but apparently he only sent an update to immediate family. That explains why people are wondering if I'm dead or alive. Yes, it's done and I was home by about 3 yesterday. I can't say it was an easy morning—what I remember about it. We weren't informed about how things work at the HSC Women's Hospital and were surprised and frustrated. But I did okay and felt God's presence and His peace—most of the time. My concerns were taken seriously and the anaesthetist started my IV in the OR on his first try. The surgery was done laproscopically as planned—a huge answer to prayer. So, it's done, I'm home, and our church life group is bringing meals and it's all good.
>
> Thanks for praying me (and Ron and my family) through another hurdle. The pain is bearable with minimal drugs—better than I thought it would be.
>
> So, I'm going out for a jog since it's so nice outside…just kidding! But I would love to. :)
>
> Love,
>
> *Sherri*

I have recovered quickly and had no complications at all. Thank you, God. I've experienced some hot flashes during the night but knowing this was coming has made it much more bearable. Also, having our church life group bring meals for a few days after surgery was so good. I could focus on resting and healing instead of thinking about buying groceries and cooking. My daughters and grandbabies were excellent company during recuperation. It was very hard to refrain from holding the babies but they are getting heavier and more squirmy, and for the first few weeks after surgery I experienced some pain in my lower abdomen. So I lay on the floor and talked to them while they played until I felt well enough to hold them again. They are such a blessing to me and I can't hold back my own laughter when I hear them giggling and baby–talking.

Follow–Up Appointment

I had an appointment to see the surgeon who performed the biopsy, lumpectomy and axilliary dissection this past week. To say there were butterflies in my stomach would be a gross understatement. She was the bearer of bad news a year ago—from the unfavourable results of the biopsy to the results of the tumour and then the results of the lymph nodes. I often wonder why one would choose this profession, but then I conclude that she actually saves lives because of the work she does. She is literally cutting the cancer out of people and helping them live. So delivering the results is better than having people live without the knowledge that can save their lives.

Sitting in that waiting room again made me shiver with the sight of cancer posters all around me. It transported me back in time to the first few times we sat there and I thought the posters were terrifying. I desperately wanted not to be there and I couldn't believe I was. Now I'm back after a year and to tell you the truth, not much has changed except that I've made it through and I'm okay.

The doctor was great and even though the waiting room was full, she put down my chart and asked how the chemo and radiation had gone for me. She gave me a thorough check–up and we discussed the complications I have experienced. She was gracious and has allowed me more time to heal before I need to go for my next mammogram. Thank you, Doctor. We asked her about traveling and her words of wisdom to us were, "GO—BOOK IT and GO!" She wrote a prescription for a compression sleeve because my affected arm was still bothering me—a little bit of lymphedema swelling but mostly nerve pain—and she told us that flying could aggravate it so this would help. After the appointment, we went right to the athletic supply store and I was fitted for a trendy, flesh–coloured, pantyhose–like compression sleeve. They happened to have one in my size and we bought it. Then we came home and booked a trip that very afternoon. We leave in two weeks for a two–week vacation away from cancer, doctors, hospitals and cancer treatments. Time to enjoy each other and the company of sunshine, restaurants and people who don't look at me with the "poor Sherri" look in their eyes. We called it our "Victory Vacation."

Email update to my team

Subject: Last one...

Hi everyone—I struggled with having nothing new to say to you about my situation. And then I realized that's not a bad thing. I've been waiting to feel better, so a party would be in order, but the past year has taken its toll and I just don't have the energy to plan anything. The other thing I'm grappling with is—when do you celebrate survival? I've finished the cancer treatments but I still have doctor appointments and drugs to take, never mind dealing with the after effects of the treatments. When is the cancer journey actually over? And is it ever really over? Because you're always wondering in the back of your mind when the other shoe is going to drop.

Well, we've decided to celebrate in our own way and get away from it all. We saw the surgeon last week and she said go. So we came home and booked a 2–week holiday (Thank God for Air Miles!). We are flying to New Orleans. We are leaving from there for a 4–day cruise to Cozumel. We get back to New Orleans where we'll stay till we fly home on March 20th. We've never done a winter vacation before and we've never taken a cruise before so this is all new for us. We'll be taking it at my speed and that makes it doable.

So thank you again for all of your prayers and support. I think that at this time, I'm going to disband this email team of prayer warriors. If you think of me and/or God puts me on your mind to pray for me and my family, please still do that. It's not like we don't still need it but I'm hoping that the really tough times are past us. You have helped to carry us through the most horrible and most intense year of our lives and yet with God's answers to prayers and your encouragement, He has turned it into something of great value. We can look back and see how He has blessed us in so many ways and just know how much He loves us by the answered prayers even in the smallest details. So if you want to know how I'm doing, let's keep in touch. Please email me and ask and I'll return individual emails. I'd like to know how you're doing, too.

With so much love and gratitude for your faithfulness in prayer,

Sherri (and Ron)

Chapter Fifteen

Am I a Survivor?

When I looked at the cancer posters in the doctor's waiting room, I was processing the idea that I'm a cancer survivor, but I didn't feel like one yet. When do you earn that label? When your hair has grown back and you don't look like a cancer patient anymore? I'm surviving, but I keep thinking I'm not done. When am I done? When is it okay to party and celebrate the milestones? Which milestones do you celebrate? Is there a cancer etiquette book? I haven't found one yet.

I think the answer to some of these questions is, again, that every case is unique. Some women sail through treatments and are ready to party earlier than ones who have had complications. Some women don't get to party at all. I have had complications, but I know other women are suffering more severely than I did from cancer treatments. I have managed to heal from surgeries with minimal damage to my affected arm. I have some nerve damage and, so far, only mild lymphedema.

My skin was raw and burned after radiation therapy but it has healed well with little scarring and mild discolouration. My port site was swollen and purple after the chemo drug leaked, but that has healed with less swelling and only a few purple veins to show for it. My biggest concern is still the blood clots in my jugular vein and the pressure they cause in my ear and in my head. It's not really painful, but it makes me light–headed at times, like I'm spaced out and trippy. Maybe some would enjoy that (ha, ha) but I don't. Apparently no one is very concerned about this and doctors are just happy I'm alive. So am I, but the question about quality of life after cancer treatment should always be a concern. When I discussed this with my oncologist, he inferred that blood clots are very common in cancer patients and this could resolve itself more, but likely this was as good as it's going to get. Maybe down the road, when I'm feeling better, and if it hasn't resolved, I'll get it checked out by someone who is specialized in this field.

Recovery of Body, Soul and Mind

A new season of *Survivor* has started. When I saw this on TV, an unpleasant jolt of reality hit me. Yes, I know, it's a reality show and that's supposed to be the reaction and yes, it's about surviving. I know it's all ironic and metaphorical. In this case, it was the realization that it's been a year. It was remembering watching *Survivor* while I was recovering from surgeries one and two that brought it home to me that it's been a whole year of trauma, trepidation and, in some cases, terror. I could languish in that thought, and it's okay to do that for brief periods, because it did happen and to deny it just represses what I'm actually feeling inside, and who knows what damage that can do! But the secret to coping with these feelings for me is to purposefully and very intentionally choose to do these steps: (Keep in mind, this isn't magic—it's faith)

1. Talk to Jesus—He can handle it. He says we are to cast our cares upon Him because He cares for us. (1 Peter 5:7)
2. Choose to thank God for another day and remember the blessings in your life.
3. Go and live it to the fullest—despite the souvenirs you have collected along the journey.

Chapter Sixteen

Say It Isn't So

Things People Have Said to a Cancer Patient That They Should Probably Think Twice About...And Then Choose Not To Say It!

(Warning—I've included responses a person fighting cancer may or may not have said out loud but may have been thinking!)

- "My, your face looks puffy. You don't look like yourself." (Yeah, I've been on steroids for chemotherapy. What's your excuse?)
- "Did you know you have a bald spot on the back of your head?" (Who asks this? Is cancer a license for people to turn off their filters? You wouldn't say this to someone who hasn't gone through chemo, so why would you ask a woman who has

lived with the agony of being bald and is finally seeing her hair growing back?)

- "Do you ever ask, why me?" (Really? Who is this saint who asks, "Why not me?" I honestly don't think there is a human who would go through this cancer journey and not think "why me?" To be really honest, I sometimes look at other people and think, why not them? That sounds horrible, but if you take into account the risk factors, I should not have had breast cancer and there are many others who have more of the risk factors than I do.)
- "Hey, you look like my Dad." Variations of this are: my husband, my brother…you get the picture! (Ouch! This one hurt. I know I'm bald. For me this meant I had somehow lost my femininity and that was scary. How can I ever expect to feel like a woman if people are comparing me to their bald dads? This is what I was thinking to myself: "I'm hoping and praying that my hair will grow back on the top of my head but there isn't anything I can do about it. Please don't draw attention to it and just give me the freedom to not have to wear a wig or a cap to cover it up if you really care about me.")
- "I feel so much better knowing you're doing okay." (I don't even know where to begin…you can't say this if you haven't actually invested in supporting the person in her cancer journey. You aren't allowed. What did this have to do with you if you haven't taken the time or energy to care to be involved? Enough said.)

- "My great aunt Ruth's cousin's mother's sister died of breast cancer…" (Everyone has a story or two or three. Please think before you share it. If it's not a happy ending, it is too scary and only helps to fan the flame of terror in the heart of a cancer patient who is fighting to survive.)

If you want to say something, here are some suggestions...but sometimes *doing* something means more than words could ever say.

- Stop, Relax and Think—Whatever you decide to say or do, take an extra moment to think first. Sometimes the awkwardness of trying to come up with something clever or comforting to say to someone going through cancer treatment causes you to say something hasty. You may blurt out words that you may not have intended to say. Try to make sure anything you say to support a friend with cancer is really as positive as you mean it to be.
- Give a Hug—Letting the cancer patient know you care can be done simply with a hug—but be mindful of surgery recovery! You could ask before you hug. I've had a few hugs that hurt too much to be very comforting. I've become adept at the one–sided hug!
- Say a Few Words—Let them know you care by offering a few words of kindness. Keep it short if you're standing. I had trouble with people wanting to have a conversation with me while standing, whether it was in the foyer after church or in

the grocery store. I just didn't have the strength or endurance during treatment to do this.

- Be There—Remember that your physical presence can be more comforting than a whole lot of talking. One of my friends came to sit with me after surgery. She read a book while I napped on the sofa. It felt cozy and comfortable. A great gesture of friendship. If you drive your friend to an appointment, don't feel like you need to talk to fill in the silence, or talk while sitting together in a waiting room. Waiting to see a doctor can be scary and lonely. Talking isn't always necessary—unless your friend wants to. Sometimes the simple act of being there for her is enough. Be comfortable with the silence.
- Let Her Do the Talking—If you feel secure enough in your relationship with the cancer patient, let her do the talking. Cancer patients need to be allowed to express hopes, fears and concerns about their disease. Opening up and sharing about what is going on in your head and heart is a sacred trust when you are the cancer patient. Some of the thought processes can be really ugly and messy. Be sure you know what you're asking for if you invite her to share with you. And just listen. Don't ask a lot of questions or give advice.
- Let Her Cry—Cancer is terrifying. Even the best prognosis is still a cancer diagnosis. If she needs to cry, let her cry and cry with her. What's percolating inside needs to come out. Just holding her and letting her cry says more than words could ever say. She's not asking you to fix this. She knows you can't. She just wants you to be present

and available. Give her permission to grieve the diagnosis, the possible outcomes, the fear, and the loss of control in her life.

- Be the Shadow—My husband was my shadow. He came with me to every appointment, every surgery, every treatment. Some people don't have this kind of support. If your friend asks, or if you offer to go with her to an appointment, you need to ask what your involvement might look like. At the beginning, the cancer patient might not even know what she needs. An extra set of eyes and ears at an appointment is so necessary. If you go to an appointment, take notes and, if necessary, ask appropriate questions if you realize that the patient or the doctor might not have thought of them. An example would be asking when the next appointment should be and what it would be for. It is reassuring to the patient to know there is a plan, and if it's written down, they don't need to hang on to that information in their head.
- Pray for Her—You could pray with her while you are with her. You can also commit yourself to pray as part of her support team. My family and I could really feel when people were covering us with their prayers. I don't say that lightly. If you have offered to pray for someone, be sure to actually do it. They are counting on it.

Practical Ideas of How You Can Help

- If you're offering help, try to be specific, creative and thoughtful. It's overwhelming to try to think of things others can do for you when you are the sick one. Why not come up with ideas and ask if they would be helpful or not?

- For example—A gift certificate for a massage is a great idea, but follow it up with checking to see which day would work (you never know if it might be doctor appointment days or low immune days during chemo treatments). You could offer to call and book the massage appointment. I remember how very tired I was, and it was so nice to be chauffeured, so if you could offer a ride to the massage and back home again, I'm sure it would be appreciated. I've had a gift certificate for a pedicure sitting here for a year, but the spa is located more than an hour away and I just don't have the energy to drive myself or worry about booking the appointment. It was a nice thought, but not realistic for me in my condition. Good thing there's no expiry date on it!
- So speaking of pedicures, a great idea is to actually go to the cancer patient's home and pamper her with a pedicure—assuming you've asked her and she wants one! My sister Laurie came over and did this for me. I can't think of a lot of people I would allow to do this, but I was too sick to do it for myself or to go out to have it done somewhere else, and I REALLY needed it. This experience is almost like the foot–washing ritual in the Bible. That's how I felt as my feet were being attended to. I was also honoured by a full pedicure and manicure done for me by my cousin. She is an aesthetician and gave me the royal treatment at her home spa when I flew to British Columbia for a visit shortly after my year of

treatments. With lights turned down and music playing, I lay back and enjoyed a most relaxing afternoon in her care.

- Baking, grocery shopping and even menu planning are really important ways of showing you care. Menu planning and meal preparation are hard when your stomach is queasy. Any pregnant woman will tell you that. When you are in cancer treatment, you have a queasy stomach. You can blame it on the chemo or a side effect of radiation, but I think a lot of mine came from the ball of fear I carried with me in the pit of my stomach. Sometimes I have a tiny metallic taste in my mouth and my stomach reacts with a jolt, remembering the flavour of chemo. Any food prep helps a cancer patient, because it means not having to enter the kitchen. One thing I realized when I was going through treatment was that well–meaning people would come over and offer to make a meal while they were here. I hadn't anticipated this to be a problem. Although this seems like a great thing to do, it is hard to quell a queasy tummy when food is being cooked. The smells are what usually got the best of me. It was better if visitors brought food already prepared and ready to eat or put into the freezer for future use.
- One thing I did for myself, and later for my mother, was to make myself a cancer book. It was a small, spiral–bound notebook with dividers. I designated sections for each phase of treatment and pages with phone numbers for everything cancer–related, and a calendar for appointments.

I had a page for keeping my medications listed and organized. I even had a page for an inventory of friends who had made offers for various things. I told them if they offered something, it was going in my book so I could remember to take them up on it! If this is something you could do for someone else, I'm sure it would be much appreciated. It's impossible to hold all of the information in your head when you're going from one specialist to another. This way it is all in one handy place and makes it so much more manageable and accessible. Helping a cancer patient with this helps them to have a plan of action and to feel like they are doing something tangible to attack the cancer.

- Another simple idea is to send an email. I was too tired during treatments to talk on the phone. My husband screened my calls and took messages for me. I really appreciated the emails I received, because I could read them when I was able to and respond on my own schedule. Some of the emails included Bible verses or prayers that encouraged me. I was usually too tired to read the Bible, so one or two verses in an email was a good source of inspiration. It's also interesting to find out which verses speak to different people. The prayers can be read over and over when they are needed most.
- A card is always a good way to say you care. Seems too simple? It might feel like a cop–out for you. But speaking from my perspective, it was great to open an envelope and find a friend's encouraging words. It felt good to know they were thinking of me.

- Movie nights are a great distraction. Caution here—if you're choosing the movie, find one that doesn't involve someone dying of cancer. This may seem like a no–brainer, but there are a lot of movies out there with subplots of someone dealing with cancer. Funny movies and light–hearted comedies are the best to distract a patient. Laughter is such good medicine. Jessica took me out on a date during my chemo treatments. She researched movie times and picked me up for an afternoon matinee to accommodate my low immune level. When we arrived at the theatre and went to find seats, we realized we were the only people in the entire theatre. We took pictures to commemorate our movie date. Our own private showing!
- Go for a walk. I craved being outside when I was recovering, but I couldn't go for walks by myself because of my vertigo and weakness. No one wanted to take the chance of having to come rescue me if I had walked too far! So when a friend would offer to go for a walk with me, I was thrilled. Sometimes that meant having to tie my shoes for me and maybe a slow, ten–minute walk, but it was so good to get some fresh air and a bit of exercise.
- If your friend is comfortable with this idea, clean her house. Or get together with a few friends and pay for house cleaning for a few months. It is hard for me to ask for help in this department, but I'm learning that with my energy level still idling at less than normal speed, I have to prioritize what I use it for. And sometimes housecleaning is not

priority. I'm sure there are other cancer survivors out there who know what I'm talking about.

- Check on the family. Let them know you care. If you're the patient, your children aren't going to come to you with the anxiety and pain of seeing you in treatment or their fear of the future. Who do they turn to? Everyone who loves them is occupied with helping their parents. I know there were times when my children felt lost. If you have a relationship with the children of a cancer patient, spend some time with them and ask them to share how they're doing with all of it. My children told me when someone took the time to encourage them and check in with them. Keep the family in your prayers and let them know they are being prayed for. Hugs and cards would also apply here.
- Make an encouragement book. Get a bunch of friends and family together and write down what you appreciate about your friend and encourage them by sharing uplifting memories, messages, verses, poems and song lyrics. If you have a scrapbooker in the group, they can compile it creatively. I have one and it is absolutely precious to me. I think of it as the things people don't say out loud until after you're gone—usually at the funeral. I am so blessed to be able to experience the love before I'm gone. This was one of the most special things done for me during my year of cancer treatment.

I heard a story on the radio about a little boy who sat with his neighbour on his front porch. His wife had died recently and he was very sad. Later, the little boy's mother asked him what he had said to his neighbour. The little boy answered, "Nothing. I just sat there and helped him cry."

Chapter Seventeen
On Appreciating Life

A Forward I Received From a Friend... On Appreciating Life

I would never trade my amazing friends, my wonderful life, my loving family, for less gray hair or a flatter belly.

As I've aged, I've become kinder to myself, and less critical of myself. I've become my own friend. I don't chide myself for eating that extra cookie, or for not making my bed, or for buying that silly cement gecko that I didn't need, but looks so avant–garde on my patio. I am entitled to a treat, to be messy, to be extravagant.

I have seen too many dear friends leave this world too soon, before they understood the great freedom that comes with aging.

Whose business is it if I choose to read or play on the computer until 4:00 a.m. and sleep until noon? I will dance with myself to those wonderful tunes of the 60s and 70s, and if I, at the same time, wish to weep over a lost love...I will.

I will walk the beach in a swimsuit stretched over a bulging body, and will dive into the waves with abandon if I choose to, despite the pitying glances from the jet–set. They, too, will get old.

I know I am sometimes forgetful. But there again, some of life is just as well forgotten. And I eventually remember the important things.

Sure, over the years my heart has been broken. How can your heart not break when you lose a loved one, or when a child suffers, or even when somebody's beloved pet gets hit by a car? But broken hearts are what give us strength and understanding and compassion.

A heart never broken is pristine and sterile and will never know the joy of being imperfect.

I am so blessed to have lived long enough to have my hair turning gray, and to have my youthful laughs be forever etched into deep grooves on my face. So many have never laughed, and so many have died before their hair could turn silver.

As you get older, it is easier to be positive. You care less about what other people think. I don't question myself anymore. I've even earned the right to be wrong. So, to answer your question, I like being old. It has set me free. I like the person I have become. I am not going to live forever, but while I am still here, I will not waste time lamenting what could have been, or worrying about what will be.

And I shall eat dessert every single day (if I feel like it).

Chapter Eighteen

Moving Ahead

My daughter was here last night, and she was being open and honest with me about how the past year affected her. It's been very interesting to see what my children were dealing with and keeping to themselves while I was battling the cancer treatments. They were absolutely fighting their own inner battles. She thinks she might require some counselling assistance to process all of it. This past year wasn't all bad, but it has definitely brought out some hurts, and those hurts can turn into bitter resentments if they aren't dealt with properly. Maybe I'm being delusional or in denial, but I feel like I have been able to more easily forgive the people who made themselves scarce during this journey or those who ran in the opposite direction. Part of me can understand why this happens. But I think it's the simple reality of having lived life longer and knowing people aren't always there when you need them or don't always come through for you. It happens and it hurts but it doesn't need to critically wound you.

Throughout this past year, I've been reading a book of meditations. It's called *Grace for Each Hour* and it's written by a woman who has gone through the breast cancer journey and come out refined on the other side. My aunt who has survived two bouts of breast cancer came to see me and gave me this book. What a great aunt! This author has amazing insights, and usually one meditation at a time is all I need to be encouraged by her. God has used this book to speak to me a few times and sometimes it is blatantly evident—like this morning. I was thinking about the whole "more than enough" idea before I started reading. I was mulling over what my daughter had been sharing the night before.

And then I read this in the meditation for this morning…

"Jesus is the gift that satisfies your soul's desire. The living Christ within you can quench your thirst for God forever. And when everything else falls short, when the world around you proves it isn't perfect, that God–sized hole in your heart will be filled to overflowing. He's more than enough. He's all you need."

Amen to that.

Moving Ahead

I attended a "Moving Ahead" workshop at the Breast Cancer Centre of Hope. I guess I'm an official survivor now, even though I learned at this workshop that breast cancer is never actually curable because there is no test to determine accurately whether or not your body is completely free of it. That's why you need to do all of the recommended treatments. If not, it can resurface somewhere else where it might be impossible to eradicate. So that's where I'm at—surviving and recovering from the treatments of the past year. I was told that however long it took to get through the treatments, that's the grace period you need to give yourself to recover. That was good for me to hear. It seems to me everyone around me is expecting and wishing me to be "normal" because I'm done my treatments and my mammogram was clear and my hair has grown back. The reality is I'm so tired and the anti–estrogen chemotherapy drug (Arimidex) is taking its toll. I was so upbeat and hopeful when I started the drug in April, and breezed through the first month with literally no side effects from the last surgery or from the new drug. But now it's been almost two months, and the combination of surgically induced instant menopause and the effects from the drug are almost too much. I'm seeing my family doctor this morning to get my bearings and hear his advice. I hope he has some encouragement for me. My body aching is bad this morning and I'm debating quitting the drug so I can have some semblance of quality of life back. The hot flashes are basically annoying during the day but when they come during the night, it makes for troubled sleep and a short night. I found a website that has a message board for women who are on Arimidex, and it was encouraging for me to hear their stories. It might sound silly, but it's good for me to hear there are others out there who are experiencing the sore aching feet and hands and everything else this drug can dish out, but they are choosing to persevere. One woman said if this drug is the insurance that no rogue cancer cell is able to grow in my body, why wouldn't I continue to take it? Good question.

Coincidence? I Think Not...

Something almost magical happens when you open your eyes to your own spirituality. It's as if you are freeing yourself to new possibilities. God opens your heart and mind to see the "coincidences" on a whole new level. I had another one of these occasions, and just love it when it happens. I'm scared to tell other people because they might think I'm just a bit crazy. But this whole cancer thing has been good in that I have given myself permission to live life out loud.

Okay, here goes:

My oldest daughter had a bulletin board in the basement bedroom she occupied before she moved out. She left behind a quote tacked onto it and I had read it many times in the past year because it spoke to my soul. A few weeks ago, I noticed the little piece of paper it was written on was tacked onto my fridge. I had no idea how it got there. I thought it was so appropriate for where I was at in my "after cancer treatment" state. And then, last night, I was reading a book about life after breast cancer and I came across the exact same quote. I actually took the book into the kitchen to double–check. When this happens, I just smile and know God is doing His thing again. He wants to let me know He is still watching and caring and loving me. He also wants me to take special note of what He is pointing out to me.

So now you're wondering what the quote was? This is it…

> When you come to the edge of all the light you know, and are about to step off into the darkness of the unknown, faith is knowing one of two things will happen: There will be something solid to stand on or you will be taught how to fly. (Barbara J. Winter)

This is a quote from a friend's blog that touched him and in turn touched me—a way of looking at life…

> I realized that I see my life as something that has been given to me to use, a stewardship, not an ownership. And that makes a big difference. If it was an ownership, and I really HAD my life the way I can HAVE a car or a violin or a microphone, then I could see being royally ticked off at having this thing taken away. But as a stewardship, I am allowed to live and enjoy my life, to use it to the fullness of my power,

> knowing all along that I will have to give it back, or let it go, or whatever turn of phrase fits best. (Oliver Schroer)

Oliver was dealing with terminal cancer when he wrote this, and I heard he lost his fight last summer. He was too young to be so wise. The world will miss him.

Chapter Nineteen

Being the Mother of a Cancer Patient

Dealing with Cancer—From My Mother's Perspective

By Eva Kroeker

The call came from Ron and Sherri's cell phone. Sherri came through in a tearful voice saying, "Mom, I have cancer." It was an adult voice on the other end of the line, but the Sherri I conjure up in my mind is the Sherri as a small petite two–year–old dragging my purse home down the sidewalk, down Macmillan Street where we lived when she was my baby. I think, after the fact, our minds tend to go backward (homeward) to where things seem less complicated and less painful.

She was calling after her appointment with the surgeon to discuss the diagnosis after the biopsy. They were on their way home out of the city. I don't remember my response. I remember the pain in her voice. I know I reassured her and said it would be fine. We went to see them shortly after. It's a forty–minute drive to their house. We were nonchalant and casual until she and I disappeared into the kitchen together. She could dare now to be open as mother and daughter. She showed me her wound and we discussed what lay ahead. Then her eyes filled with tears.

"But Mom—I don't want to die!"

I believe I held her in my arms for a bit and then told her, "You can do this—you are stronger than you know! With God all things are possible." I was not showing what I felt—the weakness and the wobbly knees. The chemo and treatments lay ahead. I was fearful myself. We would see them through. I spoke the words but my faith felt so weak. Having lost some very close friends through the years to cancer, it was an effort to try to have faith for my daughter's recovery. I have always mistrusted the medical system—how to trust now? I have had to learn to trust the Cancer Foundation and the surgeons and labs—all that goes with the cancer treatments.

The following months I had a fierce battle on my hands. Where was God in all this? It seemed I was to trust the system when I felt it was all so man–made. I had so many questions… Who makes the decisions and what would happen? Did Sherri really have cancer, and who sanctioned it as cancer? Without the actual physical signs or pain of cancer, how could we trust others to decide and administer the appropriate strength of the chemo treatments and radiation therapy to follow? It seemed like totally foreign territory to navigate and embrace. How could I be victorious over something so out of my hands? There were some cases of cancer in my side of the family, as well as her father's side, but that did not make it easier to comprehend the cancer that was now in my daughter's body. Was I in such denial that I couldn't even accept it as such?

Regardless of where it came from, Sherri had cancer! God seemed to say to me, "Give it up so I can heal her."

I thought, "Really!? This just can't happen overnight." I realized it can only happen in His time. It seemed so simple!

That's about when I had the dream…

The Bible story of Abraham and Isaac came through so vividly. Abraham stands with his sword and the altar is prepared. His son Isaac lies bound and ready. God's voice rises loudly to Abraham: "Let Isaac go. The sacrifice for you is the ram in the bush. Go get it and make your sacrifice!" You can only have the peace after the actual surrender to God's supreme will—not before! It's one step at a time. It was time to decide who was in control. Almost in a bolt I acknowledged His will and accepted what I knew He was asking me to do. It seemed He could not heal her before I let go…to let her go to the edge of where He would take over. Or just surrender her over to Him and He would heal her when He saw fit—before eternity or after.

That was His decision, not mine. So simple and yet my question was, "Would He spare Sherri just as He had spared Isaac?" I could not doubt God.

Many years before this, I had taught a ladies' Sunday school class. We were discussing the issue of when and how to let our children go to make their own mistakes. The lesson was about letting them go so that God can bring them back. They will not need to trust God until you let them go. If you never let go, they cannot make the conscious decision to return. So now I thought, "If I don't let go, He can't heal Sherri." I asked myself if I could trust God to make the right decisions. But if I don't trust him, He can't take over. When do I let her go and decide to put my trust in Him? I decided the time was now. At the exact time I decided to yield my will, the simple act of healing could be done and I could trust and relax. There had to be a decision to trust. I had to let go and let God do His work. And then there was peace.

It sounds so simple, and it was. He made it simple. He was and is the solution and the healer, in His own time. The heavy weight of the prior months rolled away and now I felt He was in control. My attempts were no longer important. I had already started to make my homemade chicken noodle soup, which she seemed to crave after each chemo treatment. Here was my sacrifice and here was His love and blessing. Nothing had changed except my attitude as I let Him do it. I had to get out of the way so He could work out His plan in His time and place.

The next months were still difficult, as there were infections and blood clots. There were unexpected roadblocks and we just hung on tenaciously and kept trusting.

Ron and Sherri are coming through successfully. Her hair is back with even extra abundance with waves and curls. It was straight before! With God at their side, Ron and Sherri can now travel the recovery road together with Him, and we pitch in if we can.

Others have heard me as I'd find myself explaining how God revealed to me how we may be called to step out of the way when God wants to heal and help. Someone asked me, "Have you told Sherri? Should you tell her?" I realized that some of my attitudes might have appeared strange to her after my experience with letting go and letting God take over. To me, I was experiencing more faith and less fear, but I realized I might be coming off as caring less and maybe aloof.

I decided to tell her and her response was, "Write it down."

So here it is—my account of how He carries out His work when we get out of the way. It seems easy, but it's difficult until we look in His face and admit, "You can do this—I can't."

Sherri is over a year into this journey and she is healing. Thank you, Lord.

Coincidentally, my mom is now struggling with her own cancer journey. I don't think she knows how cherished I felt when she brought her chicken noodle soup to my house after chemo. It has been my pleasure to be there for her and Dad and to help them navi-

gate the system and, apparently, be an inspiration for them. Recently, we were sitting together in the small hospital cubicle during one of her chemo sessions. She looked at me, smiled and said, "This should never happen—a mother and daughter sharing the cancer experience like you and I are. It's so terrible and yet it's so special." I couldn't agree more.

Chapter Twenty

Being the Daughter of a Cancer Patient

Dealing with Cancer—From My Daughter's Perspective

(Excerpts from her blog—runlindsayrun.ca)
By Lindsay Wright

March 14, 2008: Mothers and Daughters

I can't remember when I've ever cried so much in my life. Last night, on the phone with my mom, I managed to stay at least somewhat brave until I hung up—we won't speak about what happened after that.

This has been the hardest week of my entire life, no question. The harsh truth is that my mom and I both had unscheduled appointments with our shared General Practitioner on the very same day—about three hours apart. At my appointment, I found out that I am pregnant. At her appointment, she found out that she probably has cancer. The universe is so cruel. Especially because, after she called to tell me about her news, I felt like I couldn't share mine. And I feel like I'm carrying around this huge secret. Well, I AM, but it's bigger and deeper than that. Because I know what she doesn't right now: that our worlds pretty much collided on Monday, in such a horrific way.

Now Geoff and I honestly don't know what to do. The reality is that I need my mom SO MUCH right now, and I need to be sharing this pregnancy with her and asking hundreds of random little questions (my hips ache so much today…is that normal?). But I didn't have a chance to tell her before her whole world fell apart. And she has bigger things to worry about now. There is literally no way to tell her now—post cancer news—that won't break her heart.

Somehow, the happiest news in the world has turned into something so incredibly sad. I wanted SO MUCH to share this news with my family right away. And now I really don't know when we'll tell them.

And that's why I cried for about two hours without stopping last night. The ugly kind of crying. The kind where you end up with mascara and trails of snot everywhere, your eyes swell almost shut, and you make weird little animal sounds. Because I want to be celebrating right now, not grieving. And life is just so incredibly unfair sometimes.

March 19, 2008

My mom got a call this morning that her results are in. She has an appointment for tomorrow (Thursday) at 2:30 p.m. And then we'll know. So strange that we've been waiting anxiously to hear when the appointment would be, and now it's something I'm dreading. When I think about tomorrow afternoon, my stomach starts doing somersaults and my hands go icy cold. And it's not even my appointment! We're just all so scared about the news. And I don't even know what to do anymore. The tests are done, so all the prayer in the world can't change what the results will be. All I can do is to be there for my mom, and to pray for peace and hope—no matter what. Again, it's almost harder to wait now that we know it's imminent.

March 20, 2008

I'm incredibly aware that it is currently 2:52 p.m. Which means that my mom's appointment started twenty–two minutes ago. And I don't know about you, but I'd imagine that—if it was good news—the doctor wouldn't take that long to communicate it, and my parents would have jumped right on their cell phones to let us all know.

Okay, it's 2:56 now. My stomach is dropping every time the clock in the corner of my laptop changes. 2:57. 2:58. I'm at work, sitting at my desk in a totally open–concept office—and I don't care that I'm crying.

3:10. Oh my GOD. This is agonizing.

3:16. My brother just instant–messaged me and let me know that his cell phone was ringing, and that my dad's cell number was on his call display. I feel sick.

3:28. That's the amount of time it took for my dad to get off the phone with my brother, for him to call me, for me to take my moment in the bathroom at work to get the beginning of my tears out, and for me to call Geoff and ask him to come and pick me up. I just need to go home and process this. I was very brave on the phone until my dad started to cry. Then I fell apart.

March 21, 2008: The C Word

My family made a decision last night that we'd meet up at our place today before the big extended family gathering this afternoon. They'll be arriving in a few minutes, and I'm starting to wonder if this was such a good idea.

It's like planned grief. We didn't want to make a huge scene and all see each other for the first time since the Official Diagnosis in front of thirty other people (even though they're family too). It's just such a private moment. And for that reason, I know it was right. I just don't know if I can schedule my tears so neatly.

And here's the thing: I don't want to grieve. I want my mom to be healthy. And I never want to hear the C word again.

It turns out that the 'cancer' C word is a million times worse than that other C word. The other one just hurts your feelings. This one makes your whole world turn upside down, and I'm scared that—even after the surgery and treatments are over and my mom has her health back again—nothing will ever be the same for us again.

This whole situation has had a strange and unexpected side effect. My family has always been important to me, but there is no other consideration for me now. Family has become our number one priority. This journey is only beginning, but I can already feel that change. The circumstances of that are really horrible, but I kind of like this new feeling of family. It's starting to feel like the calm in the storm. My family has always been my foundation and my safe place, and that has never been more true.

Geoff and I went to his church last night for a Maundy Thursday service. (What the heck is Maundy Thursday??? I'm pretty sure they just made it up.) It was harder than I thought it would be. I'm angrier at God than I thought I was.

Near the end of the service, everyone started singing that old song 'I Have Decided to Follow Jesus'—and I started to cry. It just hit me in my gut.

Trusting Jesus and following Him isn't something that depends on my mood, my attitude, or anything else that's going on in my life that moment. It's a decision. And it's a decision that I've committed to. I'm following Him, no matter how unfair the world feels (and it is) or how much I question why He allowed this to happen (and I do).

I have decided to follow Jesus
I have decided to follow Jesus
I have decided to follow Jesus
No turning back, no turning back

Because my faith is deeper than a feeling. And He hasn't failed me yet. I'm still kind of angry, though.

March 24, 2008: I Love, Therefore I Feel

Church was hard yesterday morning. I knew that I was singing. I knew that my mom was coming. I knew that my dad would be making an announcement that they are stepping down from all their church leadership roles, and sharing about my mom's diagnosis. I knew all of those things…And I still couldn't help but cry. In public. On stage.

But instead of feeling vulnerable and gross, I actually felt very safe. I was totally surrounded by friends (and friends who had the foresight to have Kleenex on hand, just in case—thanks, ladies). It crossed my mind that my tears might be making other people uncomfortable. But when I thought about it later, I realized that I didn't care. If people can't deal with authentic emotions, then I'm sad for them and the lack of love in their lives. Because when you love other people and get involved in their lives, you feel things—lots of things, good and bad. You cry with them when they are sad, and you celebrate with them when they are happy. That's the risk you take when you choose to love.

I love, therefore I feel.

When I was little, one of my favourite books to read with my mom was a book about a rabbit whose ears drooped down instead of being perky like the other rabbits' ears. Leo tries everything from tying other rabbits' ears down with rocks to hanging upside–down with a possum, but at the end of the book, everyone decides that normal is whatever you are.

I'm deciding that normal is whatever I feel. And so I'm doing my best not to regulate my emotions. When I need to cry, I'm crying and going through Kleenex like it's going out of style. When I need to laugh, I'm laughing until my stomach hurts. The result is that I might sometimes look a little crazy from the outside. But I'm normal, and I'm living this—and feeling it—the best way I know how.

Wednesday, April 09, 2008: Waiting

So as far as I know, my mom's surgery was a success yesterday. All I have is second–hand info from my dad and third–hand info from my brother…And all of that info is from boys. I need to see my mom and hear it from her—and we'll do that tonight when Geoff and I head out there with dinner for them tonight.

Please continue to pray for her. The recovery won't be fun, and now we find ourselves waiting again. It will be a few weeks before we find out results—things like what kind of cancer it is, if it's affecting her lymph nodes, if it's spread at all, and how they want to treat it (chemo, radiation, or both).

Pray for peace while we wait, and for the best possible news at the end of this month.

In the meantime, I continue to be overwhelmed by the goodness of other people. The world is full of so much bad, but we are surrounded by people who are full of love and joy and generosity and light—it's amazing. I wish that you could all experience this feeling (just without the bad stuff that triggered it).

This week, I've been meditating on this verse: Be still, and know that I am God.

I suck at being still. I'm not being dramatic…I'm really, really, honestly TERRIBLE at it. I'm a woman of action. But

I really feel like—in so many areas of my life—it's my time to be still. Be still, and let Him do His work in and around me. And so I wait.

April 24, 2008: Mom Update

Well, gang. I wish that I had better news.

We found out on Wednesday evening that my mom is in Stage Two cancer, meaning they found cancer in one of the two lymph nodes they removed in surgery earlier this month. Fortunately, the extra tissue they removed from around the tumour was clear—thank God—but this news about her lymph node means that she's scheduled for surgery again. The next surgery will be happening on May 6, and they'll be removing ten to twelve lymph nodes this time. It will be more extensive, recovery will be harder, and she'll require physio to be able to move her arm again.

The results of the second surgery will dictate the next steps for my mom and her medical team—but the Stage Two label means that nothing about this will be quick, simple, or easy.

Please keep my family in your thoughts and prayers, whatever is more your style. This was incredibly difficult news to hear, and my mom was so discouraged by this news. She sounds like she's back to her fighting self now, but it looks like this journey's just getting started…

May 05, 2008: Tomorrow

Tomorrow is Surgery Day Two (Three if you count the biopsy) for my mom—her axilliary node dissection (look at all the fancy new words we're learning!). Basically, they're removing ten to twelve lymph nodes from under her arm and putting in a drain for a week or so.

It's good and it's bad. It seriously sucks that she requires a second surgery, though we understand why they opted for the less complicated surgery first. And we know that this surgery is just a precaution to make absolutely sure that they got all the cancer—which is awesome. But it's so hard. I'm so beyond pretending to be tough about this. It sucks, and I've shed tears over it in all kinds of awkward places already. :)

I'll add more once there's more to add. In the meantime, please remember her—and all of us—in your prayers. This is tough stuff.

I read this verse this morning, and it really got me thinking… "To set the mind on the flesh is death, but to set the mind on the Spirit is life and peace." (Romans 8:6, The Message Bible)

Isn't that so true? We spend so much energy worrying about ourselves, our health, our lives, our STUFF—and it's toxic. But when we're focused on the big picture and a greater meaning and purpose, it brings us life and energy and joy and freedom and PEACE—that profound and absolute God—peace that you can only understand if you've experienced it.

This week, I choose life and peace—for myself and for my family.

Tuesday, May 06, 2008: Surgery News

I'll add to this post as the day progresses, but I thought I'd let you all know that I spoke with my dad around 08:00 this morning and everything is going absolutely according to plan. My mom went in for surgery at 07:45 and they were expecting it to take until 10:00. From there, she'll head into recovery and my dad should be able to see her by lunchtime.

Update, 13:22: I heard from my dad while I was out for lunch. My mom's surgery went very well this morning. The only complication was that her blood pressure dipped a little post–op, so they had to wait before they were able to start giving her painkillers (wouldn't you have loved to be the nurse to tell her that?!). But the drugs are working now, and she was sleeping when Dad called.

Update, 22:15: At my mom's request, I stopped by the

hospital last night after work to bring her Tim Hortons coffee…I took that as a good sign! I sat with her so that my dad could go and find some food, then we watched American Idol while we waited for my mom's new round of painkillers to start working again. By 20:00, the last Idol contestant was done for the evening and my mom finally looked ready to sleep. She's doing okay…As well as you'd expect, I suppose. It's frustrating to watch her start all over again with surgery recovery. But it's so amazing to know that this was her final surgery, and that there is NO cancer left in her body. She smiles every time we say that.

Now, it's back to the game we're getting very used to already: trudge through recovery and wait for results. These results will determine how aggressive they'll need to be with chemo and radiation, setting the stage for the next six to twelve months of our lives. We hope and pray that the results will be good and that she'll be able to wrap up those treatments and be on the road to full health by the time the babies come this fall…While we know that's maybe not very likely, we also trust that our God is a God of miracles, and he loves to surprise us with the very things we've called impossible.

May 07, 2008: Why I'm Smiling Today

My mom is home, fed, drugged, and sleeping. And my dad is taking amazing care of her—which kind of gives me permission to relax a little and be at work and doing normal things today without feeling like a terrible person/daughter. I don't think he has any idea of the impact his dedication to my mom has on my life—now more than ever.

Sunday, May 11, 2008: Thinking About Mother's Day

Nothing really felt adequate this Mother's Day.

What I really wanted to do for my mom was to take her cancer away. She used to tell me that she'd give anything to have my arthritis, so that I could live my life free of the disease. I understand that now, because I'd choose to take her cancer in a heartbeat. And it kind of breaks my heart that there is nothing I can do to make it better. She wouldn't give me her cancer anyway, even if she could. Which is fair, because I love her too much to have ever given her my arthritis.

I'm so angry at cancer for borrowing my mom, but I'm so happy that it's not taking and keeping her. I think she knows how much I need her. And it's making her fight.

And that's really the heart of it all. On Mother's Day this year, I just want to say thank you to my mom for loving us enough to fight the way she's fighting. I know that you will get tired sometimes, and you don't always have to be brave. Just know that I'm so proud of you for taking those baby steps forward—and those small things make you a hero to me.

May 14, 2008: Step By Step

How many points for pulling out an old-school NKOTB reference? And then how many for saying 'NKOTB' instead of spelling it out like an English major? (For those of you who didn't get it—New Kids On The Block.) What's that? You want me to earn bonus points for blathering on about bad (read: AWESOME) 80s music in a post that's really all about my mom's cancer?

Okay. If you insist. :)

It's helped me a lot to break down the whole cancer thing into steps, and to think about it in those compartments complete with neat little milestones. What can I say, it's the project manager in me. Phase One was Finding Out. Phase Two was Surgeries.

And as of today, Phase Two of this crazy cancer journey with my mom is officially complete. There will be no more surgeries, and she's handling her recovery from this last one really well. She might not think so, but I do. There's still a long way to go in order for her incision to heal, her shoulder to start working again, and her energy to come back. But it's OVER. And the results came back today.

I think she'll be okay with me sharing that the eleven lymph nodes they removed last week were not all cancer–free. One had cancerous cells, and one had a tiny little tumour growing inside of it. THANK GOD her surgeon had the wisdom to remove them all, instead of calling it quits after the last surgery and counting on chemo and radiation to take care of the rest. The results don't really mean much, they just confirm that the cancer is at the stage they thought it was at, and now they can finalize a treatment plan—Phase Three and Phase Four.

She'll meet with her oncologist on June 5 to find out The Plan. And then we'll begin Phase Three: four to six rounds of chemo, spaced three weeks apart, beginning as soon as possible. After that comes Phase Four: a to–be–determined schedule of radiation (that typically lasts four to six weeks).If you're doing the math the way I'm doing the math, that means that there's still a *chance* my mom will be cancer–free and finished treatments by the time she becomes a grandma. Wouldn't that be amazing? She'll be tired and still suffering from the effects of the treatments, but she'll be there and she'll be in Phase Five (my favourite step!): The Cancer–Free Rest Of Her Life.

We're going to throw one heck of a party. I'll bring the music… ;)

Wednesday, May 28, 2008: Getting Smart

I had another brave day today. I started my morning at the Breast Cancer Centre of Hope, where I had a 9:00 a.m. meeting with an oncology nurse.

She spent almost an hour with me, and answered all of my questions. She went through my mom's pathology report notes and translated and explained what all of the big fancy words meant. She walked me through the chemotherapy and radiation processes—how the appointments work, what the treatments are, and how people can expect to feel before, during, and after. And she also touched on risk factors—things I need to know because my mom has breast cancer. She approached it so well, because it wasn't about worrying at all... It was about being aware and being responsible and making healthy choices—which actually released the little bit of worry I had been feeling about it.

I'm really glad I went. It was just nice to have someone explain it all, and she didn't make me feel like any of my questions were stupid at all (though I'm sure at least a few of them were). She was really encouraging. And she gave me her card so I can call, email, request information and resources, or book more appointments if I have more questions in the future.

I just feel so much better now that I understand more of how this will all work, which helps me to see what I might be able to do to help and support my mom and my family during the next couple of months. I hate that our family is learning all of this. But I'm so happy that there are so many resources available to us.

October 02, 2008: Love, Hurt, and the Space Between

I took the day off yesterday, and went to go hang out with my mom. My dad had to go into work, and she's still recovering from her port–removal surgery that happened on Monday (plus chemo side effects from her last treatment), so it was pretty obvious that home was where I needed to be yesterday. I'm so lucky to have a boss who's as understanding as he is about family/cancer stuff. His response when I asked for Wednesday off wasn't just 'yes' it was 'of course.'

My mom and I ended up having a pretty interesting discussion over the course of the day. I know that she sometimes feels like she's hurting us—her family—by allowing us to see her when she's so sick. This whole process of chemo is nasty. I answered her quite honestly that yes, it hurts to see her sick like she has been. But we're family. I'm sure it hurt her to see me in the hospital when I was ten years old and being diagnosed with arthritis—and a hundred other things that we've experienced over the years.

Families hurt when bad things happen to them. It's nothing bad, it's just evidence that there is love there. When you love, you hurt.

But when you love, and you hurt, you also earn the right to fully experience the happiness that comes with being part of a family. Cancer sucks, but new babies are awesome. This year, our family is fully experiencing the profound depth of my mom's cancer with the incredible highs of welcoming two grandchildren into the world. It's not good or bad. It's being a family.

The only way to avoid that hurt is to also avoid that happiness, to live your entire life in that insulated space between. And that's not living at all. It makes me sad to realize that there are people in our lives who have chosen this existence, in an attempt to avoid our family's cancer hurt.

Cancer hurts, but the only thing my mom could do right now that would be truly painful or disappointing to me would be to give up. It hurts to watch what the chemo is doing to her body, but it's okay at the same time—because every treatment brings her closer to the end, and the end means a healthy, cancer–free body—and the rest of her life.

Remember at the beginning of this whole journey, when I started counting down milestones? This month, our family will get to celebrate the milestone of my mom's final chemo treatment. But before that happens, we're going to share a massive celebration this Sunday at Run for the Cure. I'm so excited that we can do this for my mom. And I'm so excited to share our family's happiness with the people who've chosen to come and support us.

October 6, 2008: Run for the Cure 2008

My body was at the MTS Centre on Sunday morning, but my heart was at home.

Sunday was our big Run for the Cure day, and we joined almost six–thousand people who raised around three–quarters of a million dollars (and counting) to do a 1K or 5K walk/run for breast cancer.

Team Sherri had twenty–eight members signed up, and contributed more than four–thousand dollars to the cause. But we were missing two very important members of our team: my parents. My mom had a rough night with increased fever and swelling, and just wasn't feeling up to being there—something that disappointed her more than it disappointed us (and that's a lot of disappointment). My early–morning phone call with my dad to break the news was a harsh reality check, but an awesome reminder of why we were doing Run for the Cure in the first place.

My mom sent an email for me to read to the team before we started the run, but I made about five words in before I broke down and had to hand off the paper to Debbie—one of my mom's friends who's a much stronger person than I am.

Despite our disappointment about being Team Sherri minus Sherri, we had a great morning. So many people came up to me on Sunday morning with tears in their eyes, saying that they'd been wanting to help and just didn't know how—and that it felt so good to be able to do something tangible to encourage her.

Most of us ended up walking the full 5K, which I realize was a big endeavour for a girl who's nine months pregnant. It was a great walk, though, and a great experience. I'll admit to getting totally choked up as we started the walk, and as we finished. But looking around, I was far from the only one. It was a very personal project for almost everyone who was there—and quite a few members of Team Sherri were participating not only for my mom, but also for other friends and family members who have been affected by breast cancer. It's amazing to me that it could be so sad and so empowering all at the same time.

We took lots of pictures, and had a great surprise later when my mom felt strong enough to join us for our Celebration Brunch at Cora's. We made a little bit of a scene with all our cheering and applauding when she made her entrance, and it was awesome to present her with a signed poster from the team—and her official pink breast cancer survivor t–shirt that I'd managed to pick up for her at the run.

I hope that it gives her a little bit of a push to help make it through her last chemo. We're already planning for next year…I'm thinking pink camouflage headbands and a new team name: Remission Accomplished.

October 22, 2008: Good News

My mom was supposed to be having chemo tomorrow. Our whole family was kind of messed up about it—we were encouraging her to do it, of course, but every treatment has been taking just a little more of her. It's been hard to watch. But it's been harder to realize that this chemo was going to put her out of commission right when the babies are coming. I think that hurt her even more than it hurt us.

My parents saw the oncologist yesterday morning, and learned that he decided to cancel her sixth and final treatment, and move on to radiation as soon as she's strong enough (and as soon as they can get her in). They're confident that they've killed all the cancer cells with the first five treatments. Which means that she's done chemo! It's a milestone we've been anticipating for so many months, it's kind of hard to believe that it's here.

It means so many things for us…It means that she's not going to lose her hair that's starting to grow back in. It means that she's going to be healthy enough to help with the babies. It means that there's still a tiny hope she might be done radiation before Christmas. As strange and theologically unsound as this may be to say, it feels like evidence that God hasn't forgotten about our family, and that He didn't screw up when He chose these babies' due dates. It's GOOD NEWS.

I hosted my mom, my sister, my aunts, my cousin, and my grandma for lunch yesterday. It ended up being a little celebration, because of my mom's news. My dad came in for a while when he dropped off my mom, and I missed seeing my parents smile like that—not just a laughing–at–a–joke smile, but the kind that's shining with hope and joy.

December 07, 2008: Healing

Near the end of last week, I had a little bit of a meltdown. It was small as far as meltdowns go, but I feel like it deserves to be noted. I was so tempted to just blame it on sleep deprivation and the emotion of the last five weeks or so of my life, but I don't think that's fair. I think that everything I was feeling was completely legitimate. I was just feeling all the weight of my mom's cancer all over again as I begin to notice the signs that she's getting tired from the radiation treatments and their rigorous schedule. I know that it's making her better, that it's part of her healing process. It's incredibly hard to watch sometimes, but there's also nowhere else I'd rather be—and it's an honour to experience all the highs and lows of this journey alongside her. But it seems like every couple of weeks at least, I just need to process and feel it all over again so that each layer of this experience can heal before it's covered up and we can move on.

December 31, 2008: Bring It On

I've been doing a lot of reflecting this week. I'm not quite ready to share it all just yet. Let's just say that 2008 was one heck of a year...My family had desperately wished for my mom's breast cancer treatments to be over by the end of the year. That's not happening. But we're *so* close—and 2009 will be a year of healing and new beginnings as we watch my mom get better and experience Briony's first year. A year full of hope and joy, more happy tears than sad. I'm so ready to get it started.

January 07, 2009: The Beginning of the End

My mom finished radiation yesterday. I cried off and on all day—happy tears, for a change. This is truly the beginning of the end. For the first time, my mom can HEAL (and not just heal enough for them to hit her with the next round of not–fun treatments). She still has lots and lots of healing to do—and a surgery scheduled for February 4—but today was big and important.

My cousin Shelly made my mom, Briony, and Chloe matching hats for when they were presumably all bald...And then Chloe was born with a full head of hair. Anyway. We decided to take a picture of the three of them on this most auspicious occasion: just an hour after my mom finished radiation.

March 29, 2009: Happy Birthday, Dad

I'm not really sure what to say about your fifty–second birthday yesterday...We threw you a little party, knowing full well that it was completely inadequate.

Throughout this past year, you have defined the role of Best Husband, Best Dad, and Best Grandpa—for this and all future generations. It sounds dramatic, and I know that you'd shrug it off. But it's true. Mom has been battling breast cancer for over a year now, and you did not miss a single test, consultation, chemo treatment, radiation appointment, surgery... You completely rearranged your life to support your family. You've been a rock for Mom, and for our entire family. I don't think you'll ever know how much that has meant to me. Just knowing that you were taking care of her like that kept me and my baby healthy as I learned to be The Daughter Of A Woman With Breast Cancer and an Expectant New Mother at the same time.

I don't know how to thank you (which is probably why I found myself bawling in the card aisle the other day, frustrated with Hallmark's inability to say what I knew I couldn't just yet). I just love and respect you. A lot. And we can leave it there.

Jessica's Perspective: Excerpt from a Facebook Note

By Jessica Penner

April 8, 2009: Where were you?

When the unexpected come to lend their support, love, and encouragement, I call you family. I applaud you for who you are, and thank you from the bottom of my heart for what you've done.

When the expected refuse to show their faces and go into hiding, I call you cowards. But I'll still come to your side when you need me because that's who I am.

This was both the best and worst year of my life.

Where were you?

Lindsay

May 13, 2009: Trip to Abbotsford, B.C.

My mom came out to British Columbia for a six–day visit—an almost spontaneous decision made after we were already here that just kind of seemed meant to be. She came along on a few of our adventures and I had the total pleasure of introducing her to the other half of our life out here.

While my mom was here, we received a message from my dad that he had heard the results of the mammogram she had just before she hopped on the plane. It's all clear. I can't really explain what that day was like for us here when we found out… Or rather, I can, but it's still emotional for me to talk about. It was a very, very happy day. But 'happy' isn't quite the right word for it—it was happy, but even more so, it was hopeful. It's like we have permission to think about the future again, and it just kind of takes your breath away to open up the world like that again for our family. It was a day full of moments that just looked a little bit different in the light of our wonderful news.

Happy moments. Hopeful moments.

Friday, June 05, 2009

I'm feeling a lot of post–cancer stuff right now, which makes me realize again how strong my mom is. If her cancer journey has affected me so profoundly, I can't even begin to pretend to understand how it's changed her. In lots of ways, it feels like the entire world is expecting us to all just go back to normal now that her mammogram came back clear. But nothing is ever going to be normal to me again. And I don't necessarily think that's a bad thing. I just don't really feel like a lot of people understand that.

Saturday, August 08, 2009: What Comes Next

It's been a few months now since my mom's amazing news that her preliminary tests came back cancer–free. I still get choked up every time I pause and let myself think about that day…It was a very good day.

It was the miracle we'd been praying for, but it wasn't miraculous. It wasn't anything like what I imagined our Answer to Prayer would be like. We're still journeying through a place that's sometimes very dark, in the aftermath of an incredibly difficult year. My mom is still experiencing some of the physical symptoms of her treatments and surgeries, and she's still on medication that makes her sick. And I can see the battle scars on other members of our family, who are only now really beginning to go through their own processes of feeling and healing.

It's like the whole world around us wants to celebrate this victory. But it doesn't always feel very victorious. There is no date marked on my calendar as The Day My Mom Didn't Have Cancer Anymore. We're still working our way through.

And there is no way to go back to Before, to bury your head in the sand and pretend that all there is to life is right in front of you. I'm reminded of that every time I see my mom with Briony. Some days, it feels normal and happy and absolutely fine. Other days, it feels like I'm going to explode, I'm so full of emotion—wondering how I could have done this without her or thinking about how this moment would be completely missing from Briony's life if the outcome of surgery and chemo and radiation had been different. Sometimes, watching Briony's face light up when she sees my mom absolutely breaks my heart. Some days, I just need to cry, and I wonder how something that happened eighteen months ago can still feel so raw.

I feel so lucky…And then I feel so guilty. Because I did absolutely nothing to deserve the blessing of being able to spend more time with my mom. And everywhere I look, I'm surrounded by people who weren't as lucky as we were. It makes me want to simultaneously dance and puke. (Now there's a pretty picture.)

It turns out that I know how to be the daughter of a breast cancer patient. I have absolutely no idea how to be the daughter of a breast cancer survivor. But I'm learning.

September 4, 2009

My mom turned fifty on Tuesday. We celebrated with a surprise party on Sunday that totally and completely caught her off guard (yay!). It was so much fun to have friends and family celebrate with us. It's hard to describe, but this felt like a 'bonus birthday' that we got to spend with her. I'm still a little bit emotional about it. We are so blessed.

We're gearing up for Run for the Cure in a little over a week and a half. Our team has seventeen members, and we've raised over one–thousand dollars so far. Getting to participate in the run at the MTS Centre on October 4 with thousands of other people who care about finding a cure for breast cancer—and seeing the sea of pink t–shirts representing breast cancer survivors—will be icing on the cake. Can't wait to see my mama walking in her pink t–shirt. :)

Jessica

Run for the Cure, October 2009

"Child of a Breast Cancer Survivor…"

Apparently that's what I am. How about "Child of an amazing woman?" "Child of a woman who demonstrated the ultimate limit of selflessness, courage, strength, and perseverance?" That sounds much better. I was four weeks' pregnant with Chloe when my mom was diagnosed with breast cancer. I remember sitting at the kitchen table at 10:30 at night listening to those "I think it might be it" words being spoken over the phone, only to be confirmed in another phone call about a week later. Who would've thought that a year later, two new grandchildren later, a new marriage later, my mom would still be standing here. I would be able to hug her, and tell her I love her, and how proud I am of her, and be able to do this run for HER with her still STANDING HERE NEXT TO ME!

Chapter Twenty–One
Joy in the Journey

Notes from a Talk I Shared At My Church, November 2009

I was diagnosed with cancer in March 2008. I was asked if I would consider talking about my experience and specifically about JOY in the journey. This is the first time I've spoken publicly about my journey, so please excuse any emotion I might show—I'm not finished processing all of it yet so bear with me. I kind of promised God that I would start talking about it and He kind of told me that tears are okay.

I had some trouble putting JOY in a neat little box because the joy I experienced had so many different elements to it.

Here are some ways I thought of labelling the joy in my journey:

Happy Joy—I was a full–time student when I was diagnosed and I felt a whole lot of happy joy when I was accommodated by Red River College to finish all of my assignments, presentations and exams early so I could complete the requirements of the program before my first surgery.

I experienced much happy joy as I finished my first Run for the Cure this past month when I completed the five–kilometre course with my special team of supporters. Our team was called "Remission Accomplished" and we dressed in pink camouflage. It was so uplifting and empowering to see the hundreds of other breast cancer survivors in their pink shirts. It was a happy day walking with my team of husband, children, grandbabies, sister, and other family and friends. I felt very loved and supported. There was also much joy in my heart to be able to give back just a little in helping to raise funds for the improved treatment of others who will be diagnosed in the future or even better, if possible, for research to find a cure.

Ecstatic Joy—At the beginning of my journey, we found out both of our daughters were pregnant at the same time—in fact, one of them had her pregnancy confirmed an hour before I saw the same doctor for my cancer diagnosis. Our only explanation is that it was all God–orchestrated for our amusement—an incredible motivator to get better and a huge source of joy.

Blissful, indescribable Joy—when my healthy, gorgeous granddaughters (just a little biased) were born, eleven days apart—one baby was born during the pause in my treatment plan—after chemo treatments were completed but before radiation therapy had started—and the other was born in an unexpected week off during radiation. Awesome timing, awesome babies, awesome joy.

The Joy of Relief—when I had my first bed–head after chemo was over. You'll never know unless you've been there. Also when my favourite son asked his girlfriend to marry him and she said yes! Even bigger joy when they exchanged vows in July. I was able to go off my chemo drug for two weeks and had enough energy to really enjoy the wedding celebrations.

Cautious but optimistic Joy—after my last chemo treatment, after radiation therapy was over, when my first mammogram came back clear.

Slobbery Joy—Two weeks ago when my MRI results came back clear. There was joyful crying and dancing going on in our living room after the call from the doctor that afternoon.

And then there's the "Fruit of the Spirit" kind of joy:

I am not a saint. I've said this many times. I've had some times I'm not proud of—when I just wanted to yell and throw and break things or sit in a dark corner and feel sorry for myself. And I did. I've had to give myself permission to step out of the rat race and grieve the fact that others were in high–gear getting ahead in their lives while I felt like I was in neutral. I had to slow down and realize that it's okay to be sick and accept help from others. I had to give up the expectations I had placed on myself to be the very best wife and mother and sister and friend that I could be. I had to give up control of my life, and that's really hard to do when you're an organizer and planner.

Finding joy in the journey is a choice. It means deciding what kind of attitude you are going to have every day. That decision isn't based on feelings—it's a heart decision. And that means your heart needs to be in the right place. For me, that joy has been possible because of surrendering my will, my life, my hopes and dreams for my future and the future of my family, to the Lord. It also meant giving up my fears. This isn't a magical, one–time, instant thing. Some days it means repeatedly placing my life in His hands and trusting Him to work out the details. That's what it means to me to surrender. But it was in surrendering my hopes and dreams and future that I found joy. I found joy in very deliberately choosing to place my life in God's hands and trusting that because He loves me, He will do what is best for me. I didn't know what that meant for my future, and I still don't. But I do know that by doing this, I experience a calmness in my soul and a joy that is supernatural.

I felt this peace and joy in the middle of the night in the hospital when I was in so much pain after surgery, and my roommate was driving me nuts, but God gave me a song and calmed my heart by letting me know He was aware of my situation and cared for me. I had my iPod cranked up with my ear buds in trying to dull the hospital noise and just survive the night. A song I had heard many times before came on and had a whole new meaning for me. I played it over and over and the joy settled over me. No, I'm not going to sing it for you.

I still have a bad reaction to blue hospital gowns and the scent of pomegranate soap, pomegranate hand sanitizer, pomegranate anti–bacterial anything—instant nausea—but even in that I can give up the fear and claim the joy that can only come from the power of the Holy Spirit.

> O God, you are my God; I earnestly search for you. My soul thirsts for you; my whole body longs for you in this parched and weary land where there is no water. I have seen you in your sanctuary and gazed upon your power and glory. Your unfailing love is better than life itself; how I praise you! I will praise you as long as I live, lifting up my hands to you in prayer. You satisfy me more than the richest feast. I will praise you with songs of joy.
>
> I lie awake thinking of you, meditating on you through the night.
>
> Because you are my helper, I sing for joy in the shadow of your wings. I cling to you; your strong right hand holds me securely. (Psalm 63:1–8, NLT)

Let me tell you what I've learned about the fruit of joy this past year–and–a–half.

- Joy is learning to appreciate and see a bluer sky and greener grass. I'm living life in high definition.
- Joy is taking the time to rock a baby, read books, and cherish my grandbabies reaching out for me to hold them. I didn't know if I would be around to do that, so every day is a precious gift from God.
- Joy is in the hugs and prayers of special friends and family who have been strong, brave and loyal—supporting us and encouraging us through the trauma of this cancer experience. Because of their investment in our lives, they are also experiencing the joy that comes when we celebrate good test results.
- Joy is knowing the steadfast love of a husband who has had to be strong for both of us—sharing the good times and the bad—crying together, praying together, laughing together and sharing our hopes and dreams and fears together—in waiting rooms and doctors' offices, during all of the hours of driving to appointments, holding me, loving me and being there beside me through it all.
- Joy is the songs God gives me in the middle of the night when terror comes to haunt me and whisper those scary questions. That's when that supernatural joy kicks in. I know when I've lost the music in my heart, it's time to go back down on my knees and ask the Lord to take away the

fear and replace it with joy.

- Joy comes from knowing the truth of God's word and believing it. The more we come to know and trust Him, the fuller our joy becomes. Do you remember the Hebrew boys in the furnace and Paul and Silas in jail singing praises to God? These guys were able to rejoice at intense, critical times in their lives because of what and who they knew. Their trust, knowledge, love and experience with the Lord produced joy. How many of us can truly say that in the midst of very difficult times we display the peace and total confidence in knowing that our situation is of the utmost importance to God and He is in control no matter what it looks like? How many of us truly experience eternal joy—not the temporary happiness kind of joy, but an inward, consistent trust in a God we know has promised to walk with us through every situation because He loves us? God's desire is that we would be full of His joy, but I do believe we have some work to do in obtaining this joy in the fullness—learning His truths and believing with all our hearts that He is King of Kings and Lord of Lords.

This has been my favourite Bible verse for many years and I would like to share it with those of you who might be needing it this morning…

> May the God of hope fill you with all joy and peace as you trust in Him, so that you may overflow with hope by the power of the Holy Spirit. (Romans 15:13, NIV)

Chapter Twenty–Two

I'm Not Ready

Jessica

Feb. 12, 2010

I would like to start this off by saying that I'm sorry if it's too personal. But I also know that there are many of you out there who can understand what I am about to write.

So many things have been racing through my head lately. I wish they would be a welcome break in the thoughts from the usual networking, editing, shooting…If anything, the news we just received makes that harder, and I've needed some time to process it before talking about it.

Many of you know that my mom was diagnosed with breast cancer when I was 4–weeks pregnant with Chloe, and my sister the same with my niece, Briony. Hardest time in my life, hands down. I remember having to stop my thoughts with every square inch of my body from torturing myself with the "what ifs." If you have walked alongside a family member or friend with cancer, you understand when I say that seeing them lose their hair is one of the worst things to go through. It was traumatizing. No matter what, even if they will live, they still look sick. There was no escaping the tears each and every time I came home after spending time with my mom when she was absent of hair. My mom looked sick. She looked tired, and she looked sick, but non–the–less she was the prettiest bald woman I had ever seen. I remember taking them up on the opportunity to go look at wigs. Imagine, having to go shopping for a wig with your parents. Something that I would've never added to my "Must Do" list. But at least I was there, and we could make light of the situation.

I recently went to my friend's dad's funeral, who many of you knew. I sat there thinking how unfair it was. Lives being taken left and right when there was so much left to be said and done. I'm still angry. I'm angry that during the slide show there was a photo of the radiation machine. And I'm angry that someone asked what that was and I had an answer. I shouldn't know what the inside of that room looks like. I shouldn't know that they often make casts so that they can position the patient correctly every time. I shouldn't know what the burns from a radiation machine resemble. But I do. And it makes me sad. Not as sad as it makes me getting dressed the morning of one of those funerals, and arriving, sitting through it, all the while not ever being able to shake that cloud of 'that could've been my mom.'

My mom is here. And she's healthy. Yes, it's true that cancer doesn't stop at a clear MRI. Many people don't understand that you live with the after–effects of cancer for a long time to come, if not forever. And those wounds that were opened, those sad memories that were made along the way—they haven't healed yet. Not nearly close to it.

We just found out that my grandma has cancer. And I'm

not ready.

I wish life had a pause button. Or a 'skip scene and come back to it' button.

These memories are still too vivid, too real.

But if love was enough to fight this all again, I'd say we've got enough of that left.

More than enough.

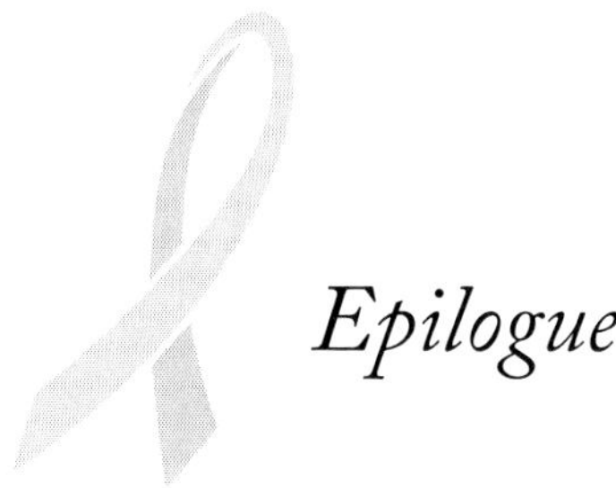

Epilogue

June, 2010

I'm guessing if there was a beginning to this adventure, there needs to be an end. Now is as good a time as any to close this book. My life's adventure is still continuing, but I'm choosing to bow out and close the cover.

My grandgirlies are thriving. Both are walking, talking and running circles around me. They are a constant joy and inspiration for me and the rest of the family. A joke around here is what they are figuring out to call their grandma. One of them is calling me Baba and the other one has named me Doodoo! We don't know where they come up with this stuff. We aren't Ukranian. And the doodoo? Let's not go there. What's so hard about just calling me Grandma? Apparently this is very funny for everyone else.

My daughter Lindsay and her husband Geoff are doing well. They have adjusted to becoming parents so unexpectedly in the first year of marriage and are loving the different stages of parenthood. They enjoy adventuring as a family, which includes going to visit her other grandparents and family in British Columbia as often as possible. Briony is talking in sentences already and takes after her communications expert mother. Good luck with that!

My son Aaron married the girl of his dreams, Caitlin, last summer in an outdoor wedding that was every little girl's fantasy of what a wedding should be like. They are happily pursuing their life aspirations in Vancouver. We've been able to visit them a few times and it's good for me to see where they work and go to school. But the best part is spending time together exploring the luscious parks, majestic mountains, and going to the pier for fish and chips.

My youngest daughter Jessica and her husband Kevin made becoming parents look easy and fun. Their active little girl, Chloe, is a china doll replica of her mommy, but I think her personality is more like her adventure–loving daddy. Jessica has been successful in her pursuit of professional photography, while her husband is managing his own construction business.

My husband Ron says he isn't retired, just tired. I can see the effects the past two years have had on him. His shoulders are more slumped and his hair is "chrome" and there are many more wrinkles than there were before. At one of the workshops we attended together after treatments were over, we were told that this is when the caregivers get a reprieve and realize the cost of care–giving. I've appreciated this man for all he has done and been for me, but I can't even begin to thank him for literally giving of himself to the point of self–destruction. That sounds dramatic, but when you see the before and after pictures of him, you know what I'm talking about. Don't get me wrong. He's still a happy guy and loves his usual vices. He bought a pontoon boat this spring and is dreaming of the fishing expeditions he'll be enjoying with friends and family this summer.

My extended family is in the middle of our mother's cancer journey. She has had two chemo treatments and will go for her third next week. She asked me last week if she could just quit. We were lying in her bed together. She is very tired and feeling down. I decided that if the bedroom is where she is, then I would spend some time with her there. I asked her what quitting would look like. She said she would probably get sick and die. We had made a pact before she started her treatments that she would only need to take one treatment at a time and then make her next decisions based on how it goes. So far she has done incredibly well. So I told her it's up to her. It's her choice. I think realizing that truth was one of the turning points for me—an "aha" moment. It was when one of my nurses informed me that having chemotherapy is a choice. I don't need to do it. No one is forcing me. It was something so seemingly simple and yet so profound. I think my mom got it. And she said she was going to choose to do one more treatment. I hugged her and said, "That's all you need to do. One treatment at a time."

And so life goes on. It's been two years since my diagnosis. I saw my oncologist this week and he wants to see me in a year. A WHOLE YEAR! It feels like a graduation!

I'm still only working one day a week, but recently I've been looking at job ads and am starting to wonder if I can handle more. My heart is craving to use the HR knowledge and skills I studied before I was diagnosed. I'm trusting this to the Lord and asking Him to lead and guide in this pursuit. I believe He already knows where He wants me to be and will show me when the time is right.

One Saturday morning a few weeks ago, I was working on editing the pages of this book. I got cold feet. I stopped what I was doing and thought, "This is crazy! I'm writing a book? People will think I'm either off my rocker or very self–centred to write a whole book about myself!" So I begged the Lord for just one more sign that I was doing this for the right reasons and I should go ahead with it. I closed down the computer and left the office.

The next morning, we were sitting in church and I had forgotten about my request. The offertory began and all of a sudden I recognized the music. I jerked my head up quickly to see the stage. I saw the worship leader point right at me and mouth the words, "This one's for you." I hadn't spoken to her in weeks. How could she have known? The band began singing the song, "Enough." That was it. My confirmation.

So here's my book.

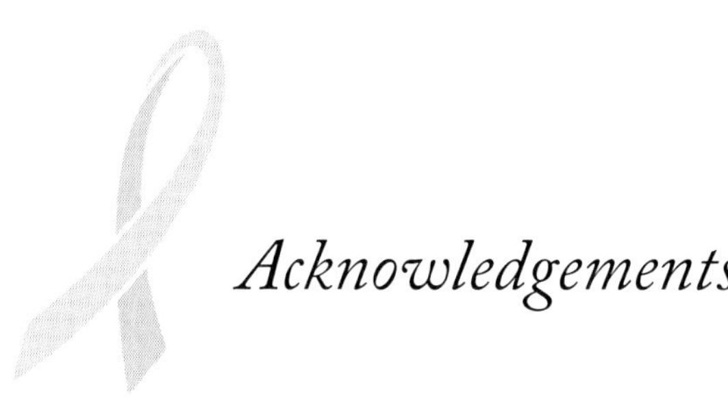

Acknowledgements

To my email support team. Again, I couldn't have done this without your encouragement and, of course, your prayers.

To the amazing caregivers I met in my cancer treatment experience: all of the nurses at the Buhler Cancer Centre at the Victoria Hospital; Dr. J. Gillespie, Dr. I. Maxwell and Dr. C. Ogarenko; and the technicians, therapists and nurses at CancerCare Manitoba, Breast Cancer Centre of Hope, Breast Health Centre, St. Boniface Hospital, and South–Eastman Home Care.

To the other caring women who have walked this journey before me and mentored me through it with their advice and hope. I want to do the same for others who have stepped into our unrequested adventure.

To my angel nurses who drove out to our place and not only did the necessary medical stuff but helped me so much with their encouragement and hope and love.

To my nieces who supplied me with pictures to put up on my fridge. The pictures smiled at me every day and gave me joy.

To my sisters, Laurie and Val. Don't know where to start—your love and hugs are priceless and precious.

To my extended families—for muffins, casseroles, cookies and fresh berries, but mostly for laughter and being willing to stick by us through this all and letting us know that we are in this together—for better or for worse!

To our Word of Life Church family. Thanks for the meals, baking, prayer, caring, love, encouragement and other random acts of kindness. So very appreciated.

To the Word of Life leadership group, who came to pray with us before the journey had really started yet. Thanks to Pastor Graham and Lisa for visiting and praying with us.

To my young adults. Thanks for the encouragement book. I cried every time I read it—and that was quite a few times! Thank you for the personal notes. I can't believe how blessed I am to be a part of your lives.

To the friends who called to check on me, took me out for breakfast even when I wore a baseball cap out in public, changed plans to accommodate my low immunity levels so I could still party with you, babysat me during recovery and just loved me and my family.

To dear neighbours who dropped in unexpectedly with warm, fresh baking. Yum.

To the people all over the world who prayed for me without even knowing me. Isn't it amazing how small the world has become? Your prayers were so appreciated.

Lastly, to my mom and dad. Dad turned out to be a real hugger. And Mom—she's the actual writer in the family. She used to write on anything that had blank space on it! Thanks, Mom, for your encouragement and faith in me. Thanks for the good times we shared during your own chemo treatments. Here's to many cancer–free years ahead of us!

> Friends are angels who lift us to our feet when our wings have trouble remembering how to fly. (Author Unknown)